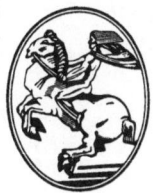

Doris Fanta

Hormone Therapy of Acne

Clinical and Experimental Principles

Springer-Verlag
Wien New York

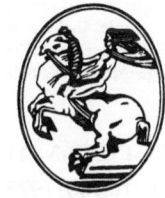

Doz. Dr. Doris Fanta

University of Vienna Medical School,
Vienna, Austria

Revised translation of
„Akne. Klinische und experimentelle Grundlagen zur Hormontherapie"
Wien-New York: Springer 1978
© 1978 by Springer-Verlag/Wien

With 25 Illustrations

Library of Congress Cataloging in Publication Data. Fanta, Doris. Hormone therapy of acne, clinical
and experimental principles. Rev. translation of Akne, klinische und experimentelle Grundlagen zur Hormontherapie. Includes bibliographical references. 1. Acne—Chemotherapy. 2. Hormone therapy. 3. Dermatologic agents. I. Title. [DNLM: 1. Acne—Therapy. 2. Acne—Physiopathology. 3. Hormones—
Therapeutic use. 4. Sebaceous glands—Metabolism. WR430 F216a.] RL131.F3613.616.5'3.80-16942

ISBN-13:978-3-211-81586-1   e-ISBN-13:978-3-7091-8590-2
DOI: 10.1007/978-3-7091-8590-2

Foreword

Is acne really just a cosmetically disturbing skin disorder of no pathologic significance? As far as the dermatologist is concerned, the answer to this question must be a definite no. The outpatient departments of dermatologic clinics and practices have a daily quota of young people who are distressed by acne eruptions and discouraged after futile self-therapy with various cosmetics. For them, this disfiguring skin disorder is a very serious disease, and they expect help and a cure from the physician.

The appearance of the facial skin is important in interpersonal relations—in the private, social, and occupational spheres. Therefore it would be wrong to dismiss acne as an unpleasant symptom of puberty and to placate the patient during this phase of life with "pseudotherapy".

Several years ago Dr. Fanta turned her medical and scientific interest to the various problems of acne and founded her own outpatient department for acne at the Second Dermatological Clinic of the University of Vienna. Continuous confrontation with the numerous contradictions and inconsistencies of conventional acne therapy prompted Dr. Fanta to perform her own experimental and clinico-therapeutic studies to extend our knowledge about the pathomechanism of this disease. These studies have led to a number of significant publications—among them her work on the influence of hormones on acne, biochemical studies on the behaviour of skin lipids in this dermatosis, and important findings clarifying the mode of action of benzoyl peroxide. Many patients suffering from this disease—suffering in the truest sense of the word—have since been helped.

Many of the advances made by Dr. Fanta have since been integrated into dermatologic practice. I am sure that this monograph will be of great interest to all physicians.

G. Niebauer

Preface

In recent years increased attention has been paid to the significance of hormones in the etiology and therapy of acne; knowledge of the antagonistic regulation of the sebaceous glands by sex hormones has led to the development of new and effective drugs.

In this book, in addition to reviewing the more recent acne literature with special emphasis on hormonal regulation of sebum production and hormonal acne therapy, I endeavour to contribute to further progress in the field my own findings in experimental and clinicotherapeutic studies, and to clarify certain discrepancies in the literature. I hope that this will help all those engaged in acne therapy to better understand the complex material, thereby creating the foundation for future application of these methods.

This book commences with a review of the current knowledge of the pathomechanism of acne to make it easier to recognize the starting points for specific therapy. It then subdivides the different acne diseases and describes the modern forms of therapy. A special chapter is devoted to the principles and application of hormone therapy, which is still viewed with some reservation despite the fact that it represents a quite important therapeutic advance for certain forms of acne.

I gratefully acknowledge the valuable advice and cooperation of Doz. Dr. W. Schneider, Prof. Dr. J. Spona (both of the First Gynaecological Clinic of the University of Vienna), and Doz. Dr. M. M. Müller (Institute for Medical Chemistry of the University of Vienna). I am also indebted to Mrs. Dürhammer, Mrs. Legenstein, and Miss Kanngiesser for their technical assistance.

My particular debt and gratitude, however, belongs to my principal, Prof. Dr. Gustav Niebauer, who made it possible for me to gain extensive experience in this field in the acne outpatient department of the Second Dermatological Clinic of the University of Vienna, of which he is the director, and who suggested that I write this book. His advice and criticism have been invaluable.

Vienna, Spring 1980   **Doris Fanta**

Contents

I. The Pathomechanism of Acne

A. General Considerations

Acne vulgaris is a common-place dermatosis encountered world-wide. According to an extensive statistical survey by Götz *et al.* [83], it occurs in about 40% of juveniles, the peak age of onset being about 14 years. However, occasional acne lesions develop in almost all juveniles during puberty, so that, depending on what degree of skin change is considered pathological, an even higher percentage can be claimed.

Of the different acne diseases, acne vulgaris in its various clinical forms is the most frequently occuring variant of the endogenous group, to be distinguished on the one hand from forms induced by exogenous factors and, on the other hand, from acneform eruptions, which are usually drug-induced.

Precisely the fact that this disease is so commonplace causes the parents as well as the physicians of juvenile patients to dismiss it as a disturbing but harmless disorder which is of limited albeit long-lasting duration. Too little thought is therefore given to the fact that permanent damage frequently occurs, and that the mental consequences quite often are more severe than the cosmetic scars.

The main reason for this attitude towards acne vulgaris is that no one treatment is entirely satisfactory; conversely, of the numerous forms of therapy—desquamative, disinfecting, dietetic, and mere masking measures—hardly a one is completely ineffective either. Even placebo treatment can achieve some success in 50% of cases [68]. Furthermore, the disease is characterized by marked fluctuations and a certain tendency to heal spontaneously.

Although the causes of acne vulgaris and other acne diseases—the spectrum of which extends from non-inflammatory comedones to inflammatory papules, pustules, and nodes—has by no means been clarified in all detail; important facts have been discovered in recent years which for the first time permit the use of specific therapy. However, it must also be admitted that none of the modern acne agents fulfils all requirements. To achieve success it still is necessary to choose carefully among the different agents or combinations of agents, depending on the individual clinical picture. The patient must also be informed about the course of the disease—its long duration, the sometimes inevitable phases of deterioration, and the necessity of adhering to the therapy. Finally, acne therapy must be as free from risks as possible, since most patients are still in their developing years and the therapy is usually longterm.

B. Genetic Factors

Although few extensive epidemiological studies are available, a genetic disposition to the development of acne is generally considered to exist, polygenesis rather than a simple mode of inheritance being the favoured theory.

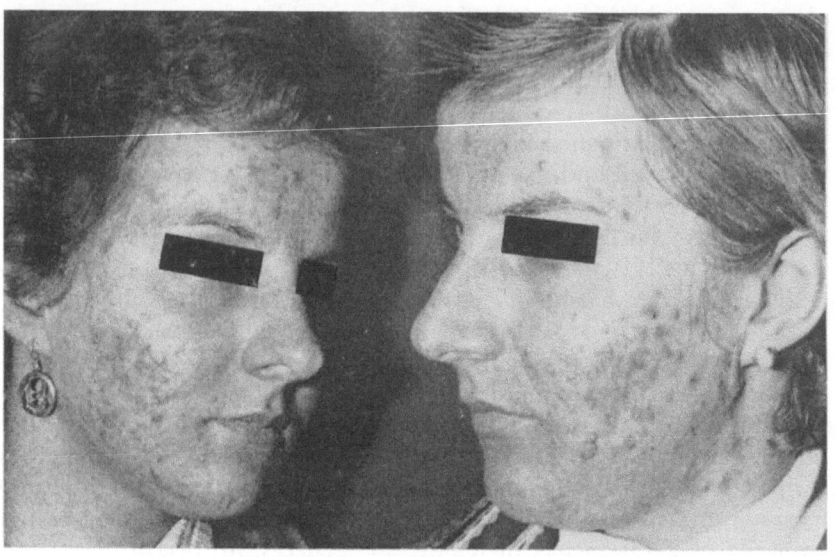

Ill. 1. Acne with persisting nodes and cysts in enzygotic twins

The first indication of this was the observation of concordant occurrence with coinciding intensity and duration of the disorder in about 80% of enzygotic twins [161, 227] (Ill. 1). According to Cunliff and Cotterill [36] acne also develops in 60% of children whose parents suffer from acne.

A positive family history involving parents or siblings was raised in 121 cases out of a personal population of 200 juvenile patients with endogenous forms of acne, the predominant form being acne vulgaris (Table 1). One parent was involved in the case of 40 patients, and both parents in the case of 11 patients. Of the 200 patients 112 had siblings, and 76 of these likewise suffered from acne. A striking find-

Table 1. *Family history of acne patients*

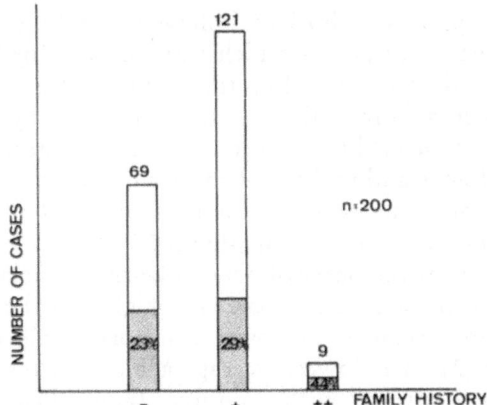

— negative family history, + acne in parents or siblings, of these + + acne in parents and siblings. ☐ mild to moderate acne, ▨ severe acne

Table 2. *Age distribution at onset of the acne*

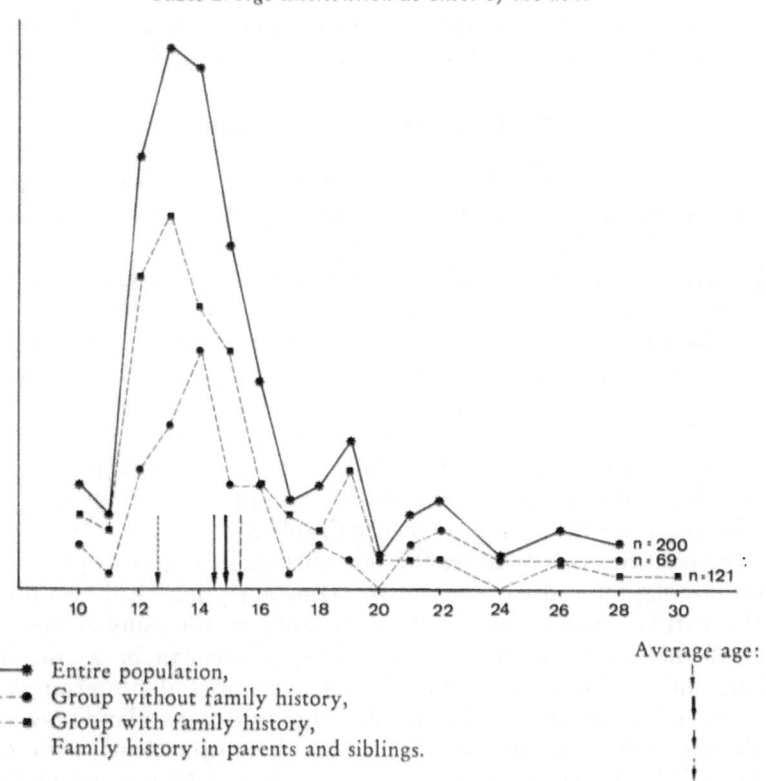

━━ Entire population,
●--● Group without family history,
■--■ Group with family history,
    Family history in parents and siblings.

Average age:

1*

ing was that the patients who had siblings and whose parents both had a positive history of acne—which was the case for 9 patients of this population—all reported that the siblings also suffered from acne. The acne—in a form with persistent nodes and cysts or conglobate acne—was particularly severe in 23⁰/o of the group without a family history of acne and in 29⁰/o of the group with a positive family history. Conglobate acne was present in 4 of the 9 patients whose parents and siblings had acne, *i.e.*, in almost 50⁰/o.

The average age at the onset of acne vulgaris in the entire population was 15 years, the age being somewhat higher in the group without a family history than in that with a history—15.4 compared to 14.5 years (Table 2). The lowest average age at onset—12.6 years— was found in the 9 patients with a positive family history involving parents and siblings.

These results indicate that genetic factors—which are probably responsible above all for the size and functional capacity of the sebaceous glands and the responsiveness of their receptors to hormonal stimuli, as well as for a particular sensitivity of the follicular epithelium to impulses which activate proliferation—codetermine not only the occurrence, but also the severity and onset of the disease.

C. The Sebaceous Glands

1. Quantity and Quality of Sebum Production

After the first six months of life, the initially high activity of the sebaceous glands subsides almost completely. The film of grease subsequently present on the surface of the skin comes almost exclusively from the lipids of the keratinising epidermis [2]. The production of sebum begins to increase again slowly at the time of the adrenarche— between the seventh and tenth year of life [183]. This is followed by a greater increase during puberty, and the peak of sebum production—which is somewhat higher in males than in females—is reached at the time of sexual maturity. Following an extended plateau, the age—related distribution curve shows a gradual decrease in sebum production after the 50th year of life (Table 3).

The quantity of sebum on the skin surface is subject to great variations among individuals even in the same age group and also differs in the various areas of the body, depending on the number and volume of the sebaceous glands [146, 245]; there can be as much as 0.4 mg/cm² on the face, forehead, and anterior and posterior sweat grooves, where there are 400 to 900 large sebaceous glands per cm², while the values in dry areas, *e.g.* on the lower arms with only 100 smallish sebaceous glands per cm², are about 0.05 mg/cm² [120].

The actual function of sebum on human skin is unknown. The assumption that it is important for the barrier function of the skin [16, 17] or that it has a bacteriostatic and fungistatic effect by virtue of its content of free fatty acids [24, 204, 191] has been unequivocally refuted [120]. It would appear that the epidermal lipids, which are present as lamellar deposition at a proportion of 3–4% in the granulosa layer, provide a protective mechanism [45]. Apart from this, the tender skin of children suggests that the absence of sebum production even has a favourable influence on the consistency of the skin.

Table 3. *Sebum secretion in relation to age in men and women (modified after Strauss and Pochi [243], Plewig [171])*

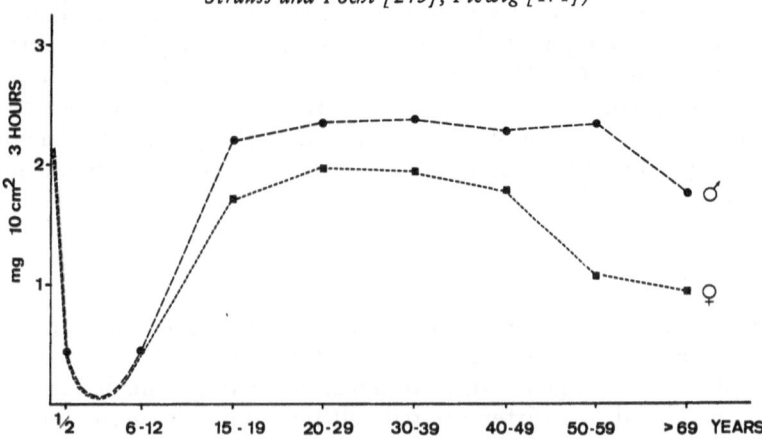

An indisputable feature of sebum is that its presence is an important prerequisite for the development of acne. An increased production of sebum is by no means the only cause—seborrhoea can exist without the simultaneous occurrence of acne lesions, just as acne lesions are rarely present in Parkinson's disease: other factors, *e.g.* a particular sensitivity of the follicular epithelium to proliferation-promoting stimuli, must also be present. However, every case of severe acne is accompanied by marked seborrhoea, the extent of sebum production and the severity of the acne usually being proportionate to each other.

a) Methods for Determining Sebum Production

There are various methods of determining the production of sebum: measuring the size and proliferative activity of the sebaceous glands permits conclusions about the amount of sebum produced, or the amount can be measured directly by quantitative determination within a circumscribed area of skin.

Histoplanimetry

The sebaceous gland is a holocrine gland, and so the amount of sebum produced is, to a certain extent, dependent on the size of the sebaceous gland [146]—a parameter which can be calculated by histoplanimetry.

The points of contact of sebaceous glands in sagittal sections of a whole preparation are counted with a morphometry screen built into the lens of an optical microscope at ×25 magnification.

Histoplanimetric determination is a practicable method in laboratory animals with sebaceous glands of fairly uniform size. However, the greatly varying volumes of the sebaceous glands in humans mean that a very high number of measurements is required to permit a definite statement. Moreover, the example of the large „hypertrophic" sebaceous glands in dry senile skin suggests that the size is by no means always proportionate to the activity and the amount of sebum produced [172]. The planimetric finding alone should not, therefore, be regarded as conclusive.

Autoradiography

Another, more conclusive method is to determine the labelling index of the lipid cells by means of autoradiography.

In the sebaceous gland an anatomical distinction is made between, on the one hand, the differentiated cell pool with the germinal cells situated at the periphery of the acini and the lipid cells which develop from them, and, on the other hand, the elements of the undifferentiated cell pool, which build a spongy scaffold between the acini [173] (Ill. 2).

The labelling index of the germinal cells can be regarded as a measure of sebaceous gland activity.

With the *in vivo* method, 5 µC ^{3}H-thymidine are injected intradermally in 0.1 ml physiological NaCl solution and skin specimens are taken 45 minutes later [170].

With the *in vitro* method, pieces of skin are first of all excised, cut carefully into thin slices, and incubated for one hour at 37 °C in tissue culture medium (Trowell's T 8) to which 20 µCi ^{3}H-thymidine per ml are added. The material is then fixed in 3% glutaraldehyde, subsequently fixed in OsO$_4$ (palade), and embedded in Epon 812 after appropriate re-treatment. For autoradiography, semithin sections mounted on glass slides are coated at 34 °C with a 1 : 1.5 diluted Kodak-NTB-2 emulsion. After 4–5 weeks the preparations are developed in usual solutions, fixed and stained with toluidine blue.

Labelled cells are counted in the differentiated cell pool of the sebaceous glands and placed in relation to the cells counted in the corresponding areas—an average of 1,000 cells. The value calculated is the labelling index (LI) [108].

Again, this parameter is not quite sufficient to determine the quantity of sebum production, since the labelling index as a measure of holocrine activity is only one factor of sebum secretion, which is dependent on intracellular synthesis.

Additional findings with regard to the cell kinetics of the sebaceous glands are made possible by the blockade of the mitosis using colcemide thereby enabling determination of the mitosis rate, as well

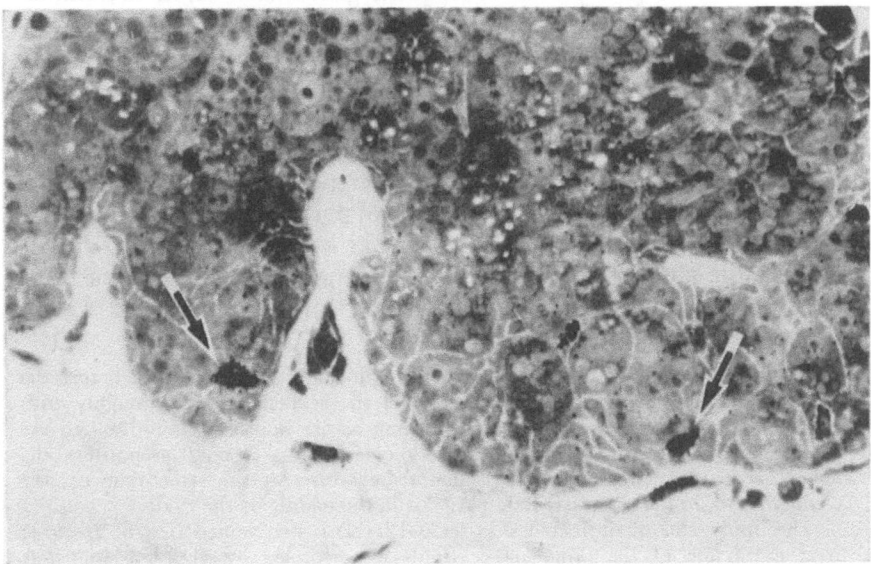

Ill. 2. Autoradiography of Epon-embedded material, normal facial skin. Detail picture of a sebaceous gland. Tritium-labelled germinal cells can be recognized in the periphery

as by labelling the S-phase of the cell cycle by ^{14}C-thymidine [80]. The direct quantitative measurement of the skin surface lipid values cannot, however, be entirely replaced.

Determination of Skin Surface Lipids

If the entire production of sebum is to be determined, the secretion must be measured directly by quantitative determination of the skin surface lipids [42]. In addition to providing a direct finding, this method has the advantage that it can be performed without taking a skin specimen from the patient and is therefore suitable for repeated use, e.g. for progress controll. Further, separation of the lipids obtained by means of thin-layer chromatography permits qualitative assessment.

The epidermal lipids, which are simultaneously determined with

this method, can be ignored because they account for only 1.5–3%
of the entire amount of the skin surface lipids and, furthermore, display about the same proportion of main components in their composition as sebaceous lipids [88, 226].

Various methods have been described for obtaining the lipids: the
application of glass slides to the skin surface and photometric quantitative determination [213], the application of thin strips of paper to
the skin surface [241] with subsequent gravimetric lipid determination, and direct lipid extraction with lipid solvents, likewise followed
by gravimetric determination [215]. The fat is also removed from
the capillary reservoirs with the last method, thus permitting simultaneous determination of the lipids in the follicular contents.

Inevitably the values obtained with these various methods display
large quantitative and qualitative differences, so the same method
must always be used for comparative purposes. Modified, direct
lipid extraction with petroleum ether has been found to be a simple
and reliable method for studying skin surface lipids in acne patients
in comparison to healthy controls, and for checking lipid values
during the course of therapy [55]:

No topical agents may be applied to the skin for at least one week before the
study. The study subjects are instructed to clean the facial skin thoroughly with
an alcoholic tonic on the evening and morning before lipid extraction and to use
no ointments or make-up. To keep methodological errors as small as possible, the
studies are performed at the same room temperature, at the same time of day
(12 noon) and, in the case of female patients, in the middle of the cycle.

The lipid value of untreated skin (casual level) is determined first of all [95]:
direct extraction of the skin surface lipids is performed by applying four test
tubes of standardized diameter each with 2 ml petrol ether to the lateral part
of the cheek. A total area of 7 cm² is covered. The regeneration value, i.e., the
film of lipids which forms on the skin surface following thorough cleansing (replacement sum), is determined two hours later using the same method: following
the first lipid extraction, the skin is washed thoroughly with petrol ether until
fine lamellar scaling indicates adequate cleansing. Lipid extraction is performed
again 2 hours later.

The lipid extracts from the four test tubes are pooled, filtered, and evaporated
under N_2 at 40 °C until dry. The lipids are absorbed in as small a volume of
petrol ether as possible, half of which is used for quantitative determination
of the lipids. The quantity is determined photometrically by means of the phospho-
vanillic acid reaction [283].

The neutral lipids are separated by means of thinlayer chromatography on
silicagel G (Merck) using the method of Erb and Böhle [46]. A mixture of hexane-
diethylether-glacial acetic acid (70 : 3 : 1.5 v/v/v) serves as the eluent. Following
development, the plates are sprayed with an ammonium molybdate perchloric acid
solution and incinerated in moist condition at 120 °C for 20 minutes.

The following fractions can be separated using this method: triglycerides,
mono- and diglycerides, phospholipids, free fatty acids, free cholesterol, and a
band covering squalene, wax esters, and cholesterol esters. The various lipid fractions were evaluated quantitatively by means of densitometry.

Table 4. *Quantity of skin surface lipids in the healthy control group*

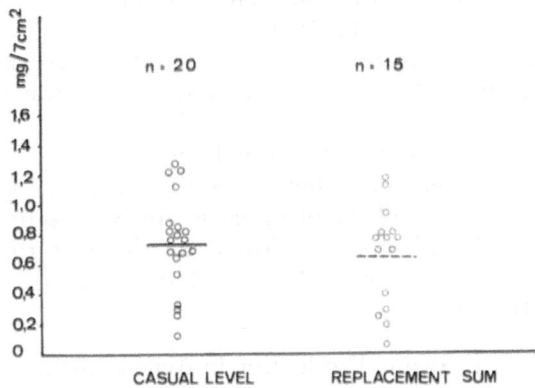

Table 5. *Percental distribution of the fractions of skin surface lipids in thin layer chromatography in the healthy control group* ▭ *and in acne patients* ▨

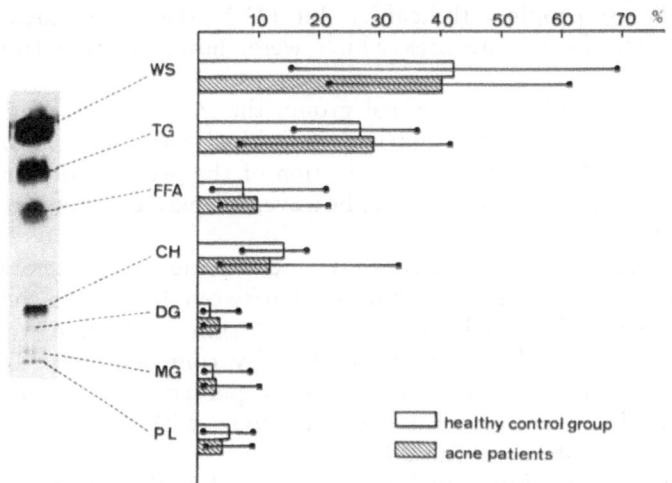

WS Wax esters, squalene, cholesterol esters; TG triglycerides; FFA free fatty acids, CH cholesterol, DG diglycerides, MG monoglycerides; PL phospholipids

b) Sebum Production in Healthy Skin

Plewig *et al.* [173] report a mean value of 0.2735 ± 0.0413 mm² for the size of sebaceous glands in acne areas of healthy skin and a labelling index of the differentiated cell pool of sebaceous glands of 8.9 ± 2.3 in the dorsal region and of 10.1 ± 2.0 in the face [173].

Personal studies of the skin surface using direct lipid extraction in 15 females and 5 males with an age distribution between 16 and

25 years produced values for untreated skin of between 0.14 and
1.26 mg, related to 7 cm². The values accumulate between 0.6 and
0.9, and the mean value is 0.735 mg.

The distribution is similar in respect of the regeneration value
after 2 hours with a range of 0.07 to 1.45 and a mean value of 0.737
(Table 4).

The percentages of the individual lipid fractions vary distinctly
on thin-layer chromatographic separation but the band covering
squalene, wax, and cholesterol esters is always the broadest with a
mean value (MV) of 42.63, followed by those of the triglycerides
(MV = 27.21), cholesterol (MV = 14,48) and free fatty acids
(MV = 7.29) (Table 5).

c) Sebum Production in Acne Patients

Both the size of the sebaceous glands at 0.4047 ± 0.0909 and the
labelling indices of the differentiated cell pool at 11.5 ± 3.2 on the
back and 13.1 ± 0.6 in the face are significantly higher in acne patients than in people with healthy skin [170], the skin studied always
being taken from acne sites which were, however, free from acne
lesions.

As with the healthy control group, the skin surface lipid values
in acne patients display marked individual variation, so that the
individual value provides no indication of the presence of acne. The
values for the groups as a whole, however, display distinct differences
[25, 243, 262].

In a personal population of 60 acne patients (45 females and
15 males) with an age distribution of between 16 and 25 years, the
average value for lipids from untreated skin is about 60% higher
at 1.32 mg/7 cm² than that of the healthy control group (Table 6).
Apart from lower values, the frequency polygon also displays considerably less scatter in the healthy group with a 50% narrower
frequency distribution (Table 7).

Marked variations can be observed within the group regarding
the percental distribution of the individual lipid fractions as well,
but—contrary to other reports in the literature [39]—they are by no
means limited to triglycerides and free fatty acids, but involve all
components. No significant differences can be observed in comparison with the control group (Table 5): although the free fatty acids,
which are said to play a particular role in the pathomechanism of
acne as an indicator of the presence of propionibacterium acnes, occur
more frequently in the acne group (80%) than in the control group
(60%) and the mean value is higher at 9.56% compared to 7.28%,
these differences are not significant in statistical calculation.

Table 6. *Quantity of skin surface lipids (casual level) in the healthy control group and in acne patients*

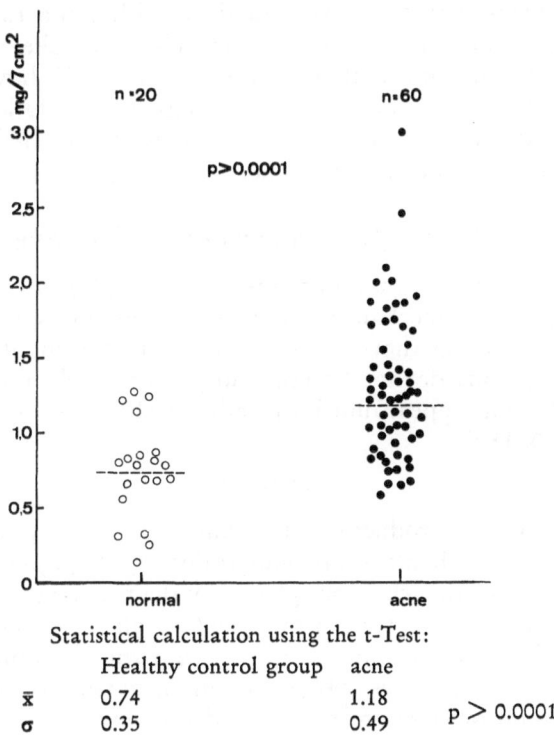

Statistical calculation using the t-Test:

	Healthy control group	acne
$\bar{x}$	0.74	1.18
σ	0.35	0.49

p > 0.0001

Table 7. *Frequency polygon: skin surface lipids (mg/7 cm²) in the healthy control group (n = 20) -------, in acne patients (n = 60)* ▬▬▬

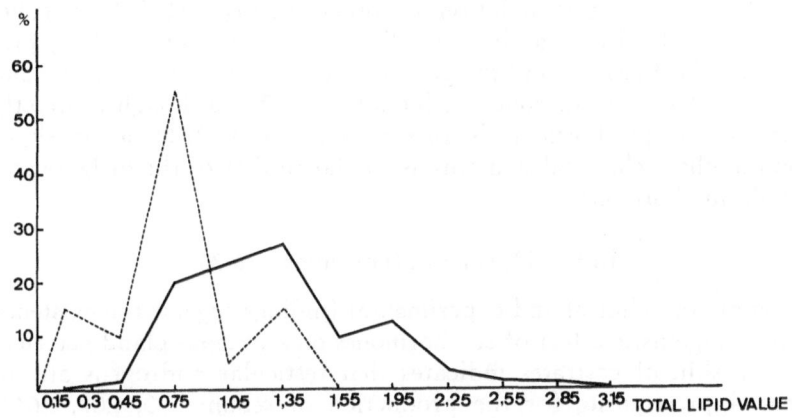

The single observation of an increased quota of squalene which has a proved comedogenic effect could not be confirmed in our test, which, however recorded the squalene within the range "Squalene, Wax- and Cholesterol-esters". Nevertheless, the sake of completeness, it should be mentioned that Morella *et al.* [151] have found a decreased amount of the fatty acid content of octadecadienoic acid in acne patients. The lack of this acid is said to make possible the growth of propionibacterium acne.

2. Hormonal Regulation of the Sebaceous glands

The assumption that hormonal factors play an important role in the regulatory mechanism of sebum production was initially based on the observation that—apart from the first 6 months of life—the sebaceous glands do not become fully functional and the first acne lesions do not appear until the adrenarche, the first stage of puberty [180, 182].

a) Pituitary

The increased production of sebum in acromegaly and the reduced secretion in Sheehan's syndrome following hypophysectomy point to regulation of the sebaceous glands by the pituitary through stimulation (Fig. 1). The regression of sebaceous gland activity observed in studies in hypophysectomised animals confirms the stimulating effects of the pituitary [43, 44, 247]: the administration of testosterone increases sebum production in castrated rats, but not in hypophysectomized castrated rats, while the administration of growth hormone to hypophysectomized castrated rats induces virtually normal sebaceous gland activity.

The stimulating effect of the pituitary on sebum production is probably based on stimulation of other organs—ACTH provokes the release of adrenal androgens, TSH has a sebotropic effect, presumably via thyroxin, and the gonadotropic hormone in the testes and ovaries induces testosterone production (Fig. 2)—although a directly acting sebotropic hormone is also assumed [129, 274], a beta-lipotrophin whose chemical structure is similar to that of the melanocyte-stimulating hormone.

b) Sex Hormones (Formulas 1 to 3)

Numerous clinical and experimental findings suggest the existence of an antagonistic effect of sex hormones on sebaceous gland activity: the dry skin of castrates indicates that testicular androgens are an essential prerequisite for the production of sebum [90, 207, 264].

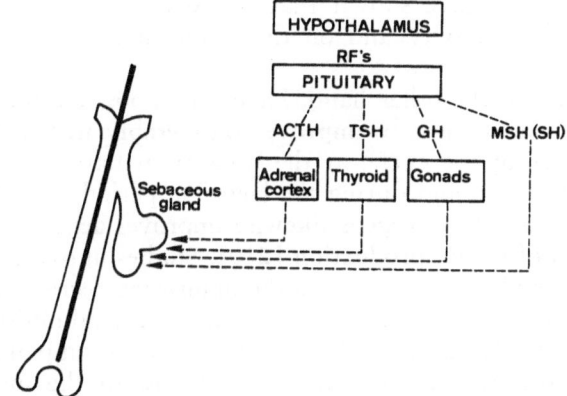

Fig. 1. Hormonal stimulation of sebum production [by Winkler (269)]

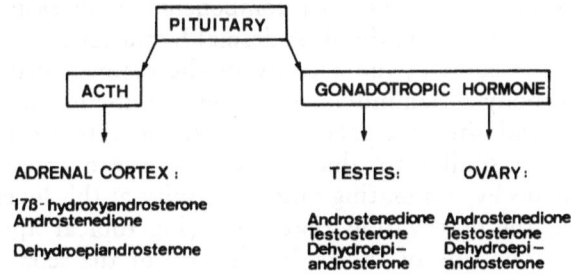

Fig. 2. Pituitary regulation of androgen production

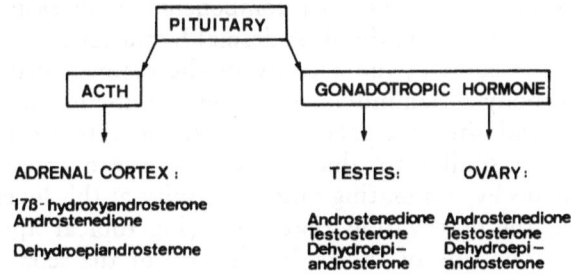

Formulas 1—3

Furthermore, the picture of seborrhoea and acne can frequently be observed in androgen-producing, virilizing tumours, e.g. arrheno-blastoma, hilus cell tumour, lipoid cell tumour, and adrenal hyper-plasia, and under the therapeutic administration of androgens, e.g. in children with cryptorchism and in mammary carcinoma.

Studies in rats have shown that androgens have a stimulatory effect on mitotic activity and on the intracellular synthesis of lipids [51, 91].

Oestrogens, on the other hand, have the opposite effect: existing seborrhoea and acne usually improve considerably in the oestrogen-dominant phase of the cycle, at the time of ovulation, in the later phases of pregnancy, and during the lactation period. The therapeutic administration of oestrogens likewise improves acne via a significant reduction of sebum production [210]. Studies in ovariectomized, testosterone-stimulated rats confirm the significant decrease in sebaceous gland volume following systemic and topical administration of oestrogens [41, 101, 201]. This is not, however, accompanied by the decreased mitosis rate in the sebaceous glands, so the main target for the inhibitory effect of oestrogens is probably the intracellular synthesis of lipids [40].

In addition to sebaceous gland inhibition, oestrogens are known to have various effects on numerous components of the skin [222]. For instance, the increased synthesis of dermal hyaluronic acid leads to an increased water content, the activity of the pigment cells in various areas of the body—mammillae, perineum—is increased. Depending on the dose and site oestrogens can exert an antimitotic and anti-synthetic effect similar to glucocorticoids, or can cause thickening of the epidermis by stimulating mitotic activity at this level [195].

Based on the observation that, following topical application of oestrogens to one side of the body, the size of the sebaceous glands diminished on the untreated side as well [236, 269], it was concluded that oestrogens have a primarily central mechanism of action via inhibition of gonadotropin secretion and, hence, inhibition of androgen production. Studies in castrated rabbits, however, have proved that oestrogens also have a local effect [256]: sebaceous gland hyperplasia induced by the administration of androgens can be suppressed by the topical use of oestrogens at the site of application. Furthermore, when oestrogens are administered beforehand, sebum production is not stimulated by topical application of testosterone—further evidence for a topical effect of oestrogens.

Although acne in the female was initially attributed to the effect of adrenal androgens, the absence of acne in castrates and females with ovarian dysfunction [208] indicated that the adrenal androgens alone are not sufficient explanation. It was also observed that acne in the female tends to deteriorate precisely in the two phases in which elevated progesterone levels are present, i.e. in the luteal phase of the cycle and at the beginning of pregnancy [6, 235]. Parallel to the progesterone variations, various authors also observe fluctuating values for skin surface lipids [112, 261]: about 50% of females display a characteristic curve for the skin surface lipids corresponding to the cycle pattern, with low preovulatory values, an increase at mid-cycle and high postovulatory values [92].

Progesterone exhibits a similar androgenic effect to testosterone in studies in oophorectomised rats [93]. Moreover, seborrhoea has been induced experimentally in females with healthy skin by means of 3 months' administration of 30–50 mg progesterone/day—i.e. doses which approximate the amounts produced in the luteal phase, and was found to be reversible after discontinuation of the progesterone medication [6, 178, 280]. The changes were particularly pronounced when progesterone was administered only in the premenstrual phase, presumably because of accentuation of the physiological effect [280].

The spectrum of action of progestogens is, however, extremely diverse due to the fact that progesterone is a central intermediate product in the biosynthesis of all other sex steroids. Some progestogens, for example, have an additional oestrogenic or pronounced androgenic concomitant effect. Finally, an antigonadotropic effect can generally be expected at high doses [21].

Thus, the activity of the sebaceous glands is subject to extremely complex hormonal regulation. Only rarely, however, are increased sebaceous gland activity and the subsequently appearing acne lesions the symptom of an underlying over-production of androgens. No detectable endocrinological disorders are present in the overwhelming majority of cases.

Androgen Values in Acne Patients

The reports so far published in the literature on the serum and urinary androgen levels in acne patients are highly contradictory: while some authors observe completely normal androgen values [179], others report cases of elevated serum testosterone values in comparison to healthy controls [130, 126], although the control groups in the study series involving male patients were not reliably matched to the stage of development of the patient groups. Elevated serum testosterone values have been reported in 30–45% of an unselected population of female patients [66, 144], while cases of elevated 17-β-hydroxysteroids and increased androstanediol elimination have also been observed [42, 134, 141]. An increased production of adrenal and ovarian androgens has also been induced in some of the patients by stimulation with ACTH or HCG.

Serum testosterone values were determined by means of radioimmunoassay in an extensive, unselected population of 180 female patients (age distribution between 15 and 39 years) who presented at our outpatient department with acne (Table 8) [60].

An antiserum displaying a 100% cross reaction with dihydrotestosterone (DHT) is used to determine serum testosterone. Consequently, celite column chromatography is first of all performed to separate the DHT following ether extraction of the serum. Subsequent incubation for the radioimmunological determination is performed according to the method described [75], dextranecoated animal charcoal being used to separate the free from the bound tracer. The data were evaluated by a computer program [231].

Table 8. *Serum testosterone values in acne patients (n = 180), mean value: 38 ng/ml*

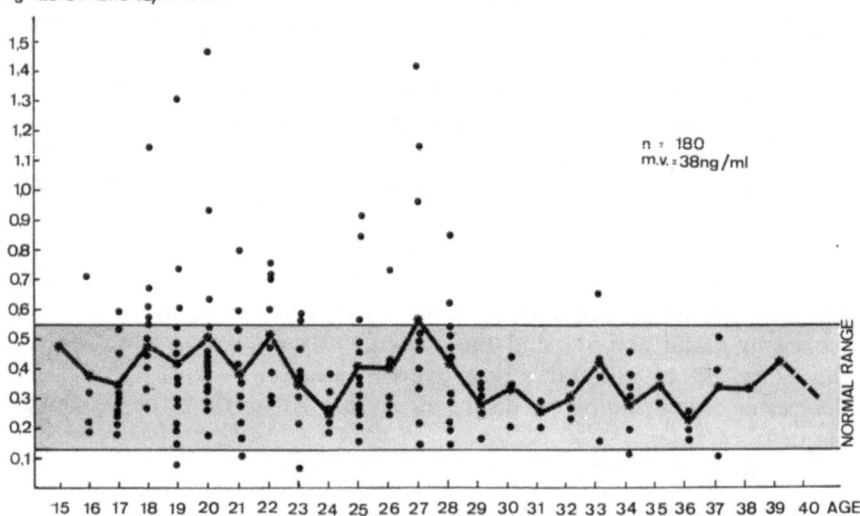

ng TESTOSTERONE/ml serum

The mean value for serum testosterone in the population studied—0.38 ng/ml—is well within the normal range (0.13–0.55), if slightly above the mean value of the latter (0.21). No differences can be recognized between serum testosterone levels in pubertal and post-pubertal acne. The serum testosterone values are distinctly to greatly increased in only 30 cases—17%.

These results permit the conclusion that, in a fairly large population of female acne patients, one must always expect to find a certain percentage of cases in which the acne must be regarded as a symptom of elevated serum androgen levels and which require further endocrinological clarification. In the overwhelming majority of cases, however, the situation is completely normal. Thus, although elevated androgen levels must be expected to have a promoting effect on the development of acne, they should not be regarded as a prerequisite.

c) Androgen Metabolism of the Skin

The skin is not, however, only a receptor of androgenic stimuli—as in the prostate and testes, androgen metabolism of varying intensity takes place in all areas of the skin [74, 206, 265, 275]. A major step in this respect is the formation of dihydrotestosterone (DHT), a potent metabolite with respect to growth stimulation of the terminal organ [61, 264]. DHT derives from testosterone [82] and, in the female, from androstenedione as well [141].

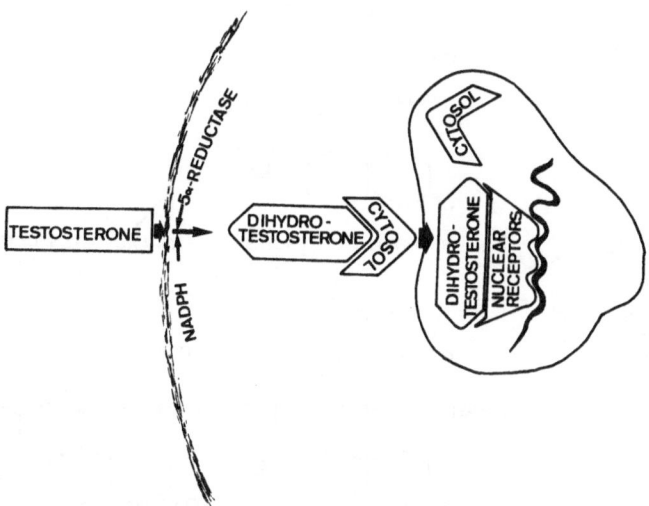

Fig. 3. Presumed testosterone metabolism in the target organ

The hypothesis exists that the production of DHT increases in special regions of the skin in a genetically determined rhythm. For example, the conversion of vellus hair into terminal hair is attributed to increased DHT metabolism at certain hair follicles at the time of puberty. Apart from the physiological change, however, the same process can also cause undesired effects, e.g. acne, hirsutism, and androgenic effluvium [185].

The enzyme 5-α-reductase plays a major role in the conversion of testosterone to DHT [254]. The fact that the main part of this enzyme's activity is bound to microsomes has led to the belief that free testosterone or androstenedione penetrates into the cell of the target organs, is reduced there by means of 5-α-reductase in the presence of the cofactor nicotinamide adenine dinucleotide phosphate (NADPH) in the microsomes [253], is then bound to a specific receptor protein—cytosol [103]—and is then transported into the cell

nucleus as an activated protein-hormone complex [18]. This androgen receptor likewise appears to be particularly important for the
development of seborrhoea or acne lesions, since it has so far been
demonstrated only in seborrhoeic skin, and never in healthy skin [19].
In the cell nucleus the hormone is transferred to a nuclear receptor,
which passes it on to the chromatin substance, where transcription

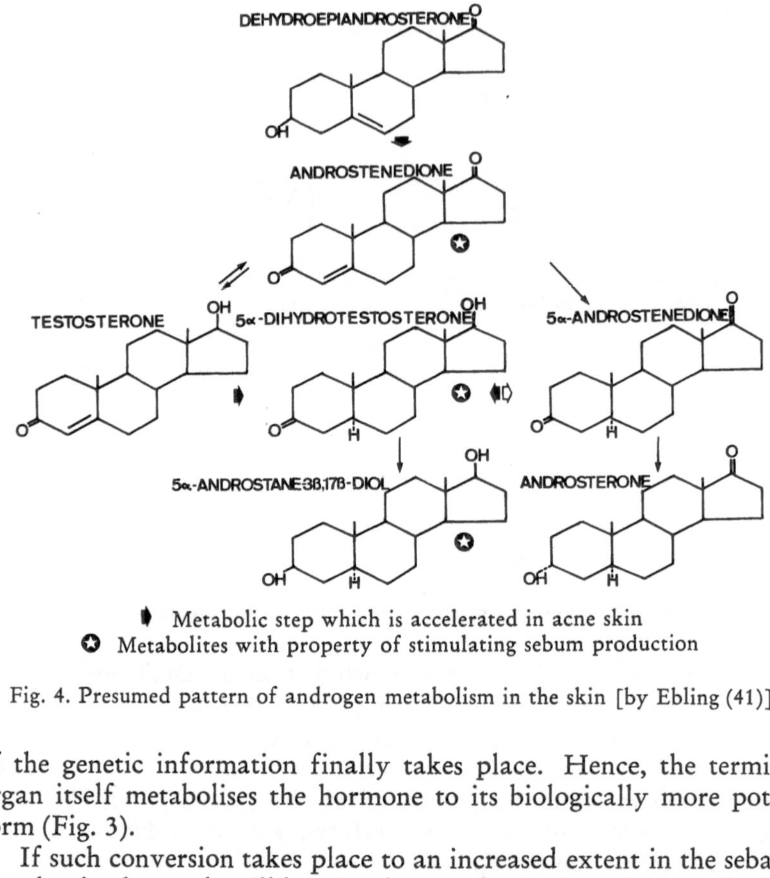

♦ Metabolic step which is accelerated in acne skin
✪ Metabolites with property of stimulating sebum production

Fig. 4. Presumed pattern of androgen metabolism in the skin [by Ebling (41)]

of the genetic information finally takes place. Hence, the terminal
organ itself metabolises the hormone to its biologically more potent
form (Fig. 3).

     If such conversion takes place to an increased extent in the sebace-
ous glands, the result will be stimulation of mitotic activity and of the
intracellular synthesis of lipids and, hence, stimulation of sebum production. DHT concentrations up to 20 times higher than in healthy
subjects of the same age group have, in fact, been observed in the
skin of acne patients, although regional differences with higher values
in the typical acne areas can also be observed [94, 141, 212]. It has
recently been reported that, in acne skin, dehydroepiandrosterone is
also metabolized at an increased rate to androstenedione—which

also displays a stimulatory effect on sebaceous glands in animal experiments—via a 3-β-hydroxy-steroid-dehydrogenase 4-5-isomerase. Finally, androstanediol, a degradation product of DHT which is eliminated in increased amounts in the urine of acne patients [141], probably also has a stimulatory effect on the sebaceous glands and must therefore be partly responsible for the development of seborrhoea (Fig. 4).

Pharmacological studies in rats have shown that the formation of DHT is subject to pituitary control [44]—the "sebotropic" hormone appears to influence the formation and activation of the enzyme 5-α-reductase and the nuclear and cytoplasmic receptor proteins.

Whether increased sebum production alone or a DHT-dependent change in the thickness and keratin quality or permeability of the follicular epithelium as well results from the increased formation of DHT has not yet been fully clarified.

Histochemical studies with demonstration of dehydrogenases have led to a localization of testosterone metabolism in small areas of the acini and excretory ducts of sebaceous glands, and it can be assumed that it is here where the increased androgenic effect then leads to an increase of the mitosis rate and thus to seborrhoea and increased epithelial proliferation [27].

D. The Follicular Epithelium

1. Pathological Keratinization

Disturbed hornification develops in special, probably genetic sensitivity of the follicular epithelium partly as a result of a direct influence of hormonal factors and partly, it is presumed, via induction by proliferationactivating components of the follicular contents—sebum displays a stimulatory effect on keratinizing epithelia in animal experiments.

At first, histological and autioradiographic studies led to the assumption of an increased mitosis rate of keratinocytes with an increased production of horny substance [176].

In addition to the quantitative change, however, there are also qualitative differences: whereas a granulosa layer is present in the upper part—the acroinfundibulum—of the healthy follicle, it is missing under normal conditions in the lower part, the infrainfundibulum. Only flat, loosely flaking horny cells which transport the stream of sebum to the surface are produced here. In the microcomedo, the preceeding stage of a comedo, which is regarded as the primary manifestation of acne vulgaris, a granulosa layer also occurs

2*

in the infrainfundibulum. Solid, interconnected horny lamellae are now formed here [176, 186]. Thus, an increased amount of keratin is produced which hardly scales off because of the compact connection of the cells—analogous to retention hyperkeratosis [170] (Ill. 3 a–c).

The granulosa layer of the microcomedo in the infrainfundibulum differs under the electron microscope from that of the epidermis by virtue of distinct thickening of the cell membranes, a lower number of tonofilaments, and an accumulation of enlarged keratohyalin granula [124]. Since the horny cells are normally separated by enzymatic action, the reason for the solid adhesion of the cells obtaining here might be that the thickened cell membranes are more resistant or that the enzymatic mechanism is disturbed.

The Odland bodies—organelles deposited intracytoplasmatically in the upper layers of keratinizing epithelia—are distinctly reduced in comedonal epithelium. It has not yet been clarified whether they bring about normal desquamation by means of their content of hydrolytic enzymes [255, 271] or whether the substances in them, which can be demonstrated by means of the osmium-zinc-iodide technique and which presumably correspond to lipoproteins, play a role in keratinization [159].

Drops of incorporated lipid can be demonstrated in the cells of the granulosa layer of the comedonal epithelium, which indicates that the process of pathological hornification begins beneath the keratin layer. Absorption of sebaceous gland lipids is unlikely. Either the cells produce abnormal lipids, or the enzymes which under normal conditions break down the lipids are absent, or modified keratin is produced which cannot combine with the normal lipids. The occasional incorporation of lipids in psoriatic scales, for example, are also attributed to the last mechanism [140].

Horny lamellae and incorporated sebum distend the follicular infundibulum. The pore dilates if the process also affects the acroinfundibulum, resulting in the well-known picture of the open comedo with the melanin-stained blackish-brown plug (Ill. 4). If the acroinfundibulum remains unaffected, the "closed" comedo with a follicular opening visible only under the microscope develops on further cystic dilatation (Ill. 5). Closed and open comedones are the source of the following inflammations [165].

2. Lysis and Inflammatory Reaction

At first it was thought that the epithelium ruptures primarily as a result of injurious influences from inside the follicle—pressure of sebum and horny masses, degradation products of the sebum—and

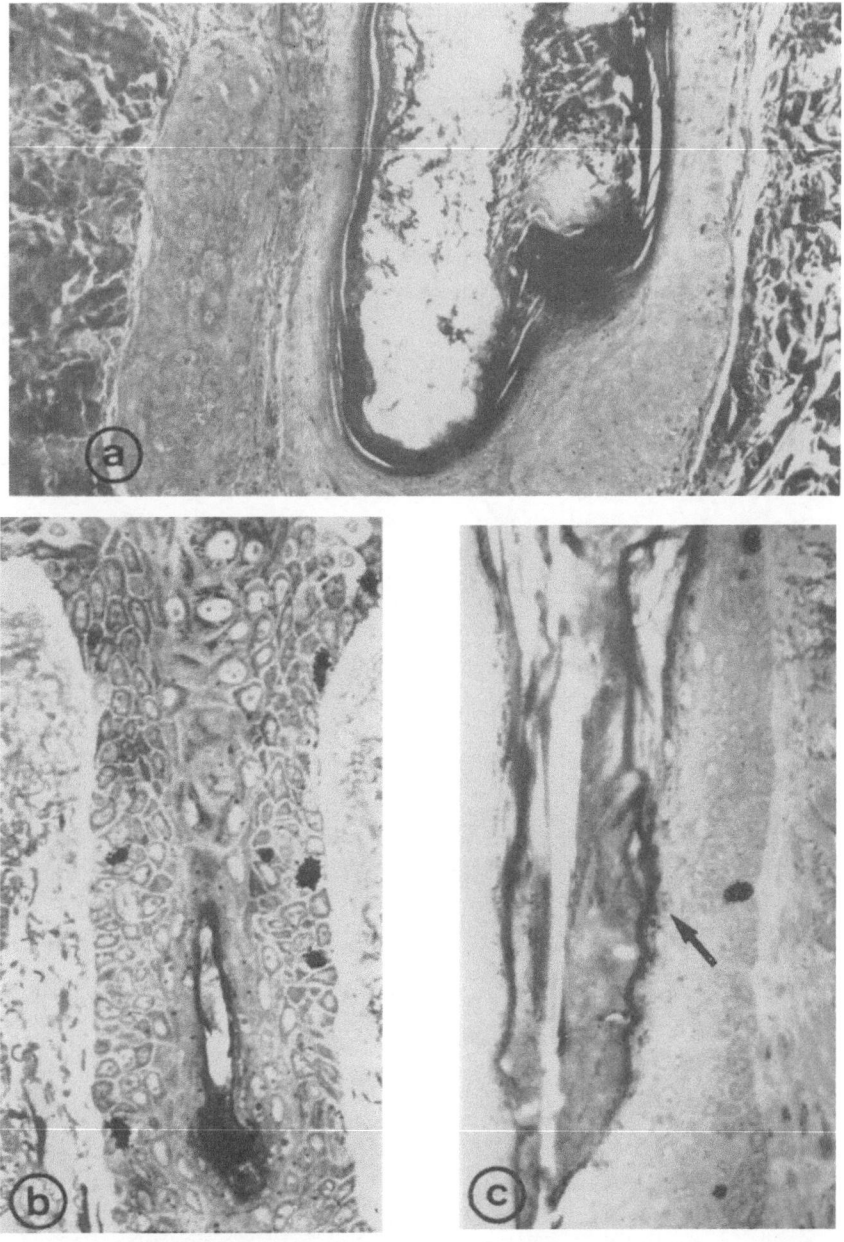

Ill. 3. *a* Methylene blue-stained Epon-semithin section. Facial skin, comedonal acne. Suprasseboglandular section of the follicular infundibulum (×310), *b*, *c* autoradiography of Epon-embedded material, facial skin, comedonal acne (×400), *b* incipient formation of comedones, *c* the stratum granulosum is very pronounced in this section of the follicle (→)

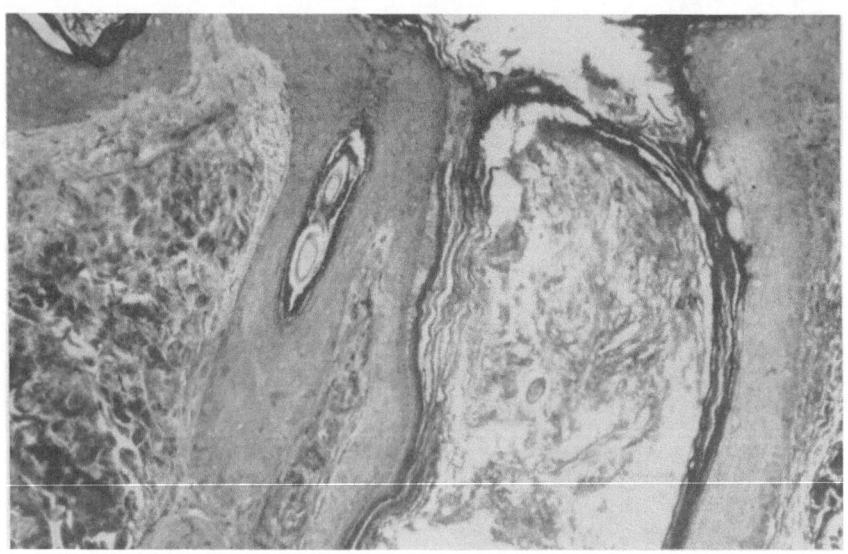

Ill. 4. Methylene blue-stained Epon semithin section. Open comedo ($\times$160)

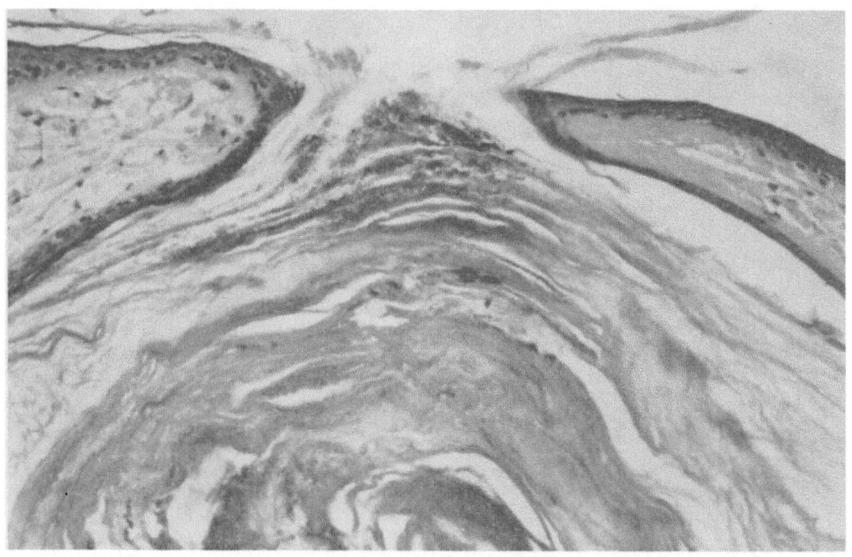

Ill. 5. HE-stained paraffin section. "Closed" comedo ($\times$310)

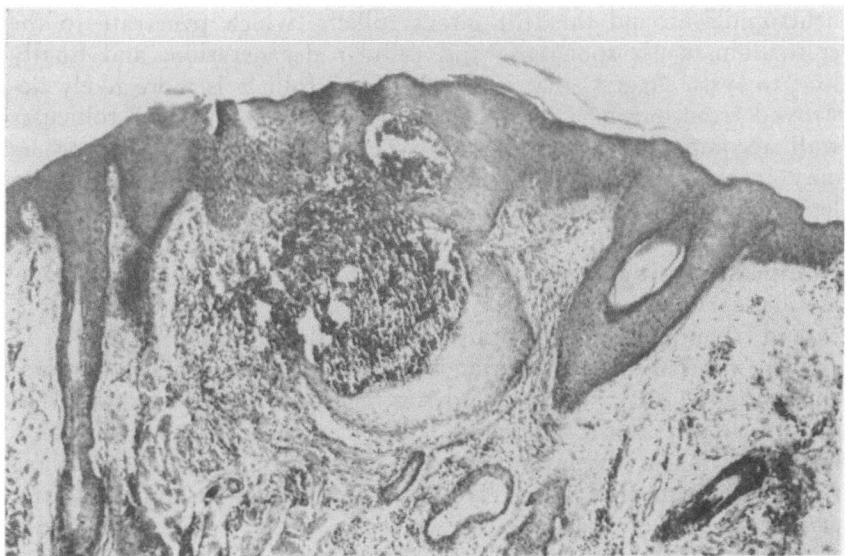

Ill. 6. HE-stained paraffin section. Acne papule (×80)

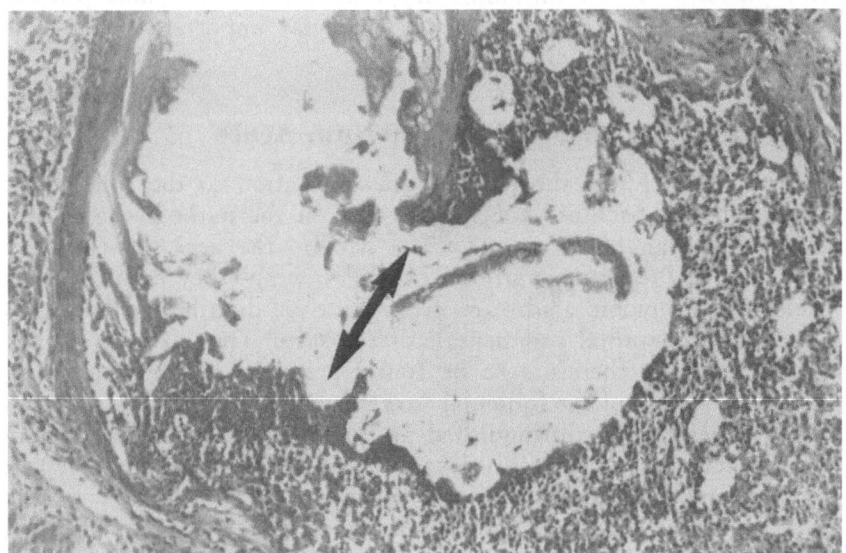

Ill. 7. HE-stained paraffin section. Rupture of the follicular wall

that the subsequent emergence of the contents of the follicle is the cause of an inflammatory process. However, the accumulation of neutrophils around the still intact follicle, which penetrate to the epithelium, cause spongiosis and cellular degeneration, and finally lead to lysis, suggests that the wall of the follicle is more likely destroyed from outside [119]. Apart from this, lysis of the follicular wall accompanied by inflammatory reactions by no means occurs only in the damaged wall of comedones, but also—although to a lesser extent—in follicles of normal appearance [239].

Thus, although the cause of destroyance of the follicular wall is still unknown, it appears to be certain that the extent of the inflammation correlates with that of the deluscence and that the lesions extend from quickly healing pustules to persisting nodes (Ill. 6, 7).

The experimental intracutaneous application of sebum and comedo content [238], which led to severe inflammatory reactions, has shown that it is the emerging follicular content which provokes intensification of the inflammatory infiltrate following lysis. These reactions are particularly severe after injection of insoluble keratin, giant cells also occurring as an expression of the foreign body reaction [194].

It is obvious from the processes described above that acne papules and pustules are an inflammatory and not an infectious process; despite this, a microorganism is of particular importance in the development of acne lesions.

E. Propionibacterium Acnes

Unna [251] was the first to draw attention to the role of the "bottle-shaped bacillus" corynebacterium in the pathomechanism of acne more than 80 years ago. The bacilli—the new nomenclature for which is *Propionibacterium acnes* (*P. acnes*)—they convert lactic acids into propionic acid—are gram-positive, diphtheroid rods and belong to the normal commensals of the skin. They are strictly anaerobic and are therefore to be found primarily in the suprasebo-glandular section of the follicular excretory duct.

P. acnes can be distinguished as type 1 from the metabolically more potent but considerably less frequent propionibacterium type 2 or propionibacterium granulosum by means of morphology of the colonies, phage sensitivity, biochemical reactions, and immunological specificity.

An initial, major indication of the pathogenetic importance of *P. acnes* in acne was its more frequent, more regular, and more numerous occurrence in acne lesions in comparison to the other commensals of the follicles—the staphylococci and *Pityrosporon ovale* [106, 147, 224, 229]. Extensive lagoons of *P. acnes* with 10^4–10^7 germs per follicle can be found in every microcomedo (Ill. 8).

The age distribution curve runs virtually parallel to that of sebum production: they are hardly ever encountered before puberty, since survival conditions are poor without an adequate sebum production;

Tabelle 9. *Red fluorescence of facial skin due to porphyrins produced by propionibacterium acnes. Age distribution [by Bues (22)]*

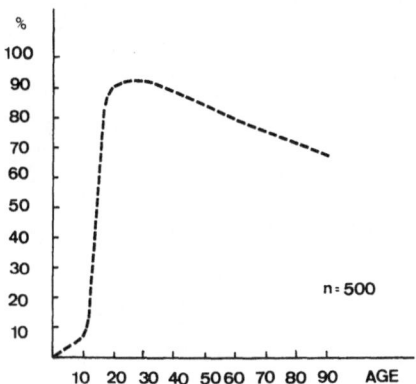

from the 16th year of life onwards, however, they occur at a density of about 600 germs/cm² skin surface, and even achieve values of up to 85,000 germs/cm² in acne patients [133] (Table 9).

A few other factors suggest that *P. acnes* promotes the genesis of comedones and is co-responsible for the subsequent inflammatory changes: lipid extracts of *P. acnes* have been found to be comedogenic in experiments on the rabbit ear. Injections of *P. acnes* suspensions into the sterile contents of the steatocystoma multiplex led to inflammation, whereas coccal suspensions provoked no reactions at all [44]. Finally exogenous comedones induced by tar and oil, which contain only small amounts of *P. acnes,* are followed much less frequently by inflammatory reactions.

1. Enzymatic Activity

As already mentioned, acne should by no means be regarded as a bacterial infection, nor is *P. acnes* the sole pathogenic agent. In fact, modern opinion is that *P. acnes* plays more of an indirect role via metabolic products and biochemical changes of the sebum: the enzymatic activity of *P. acnes* is extremely high.

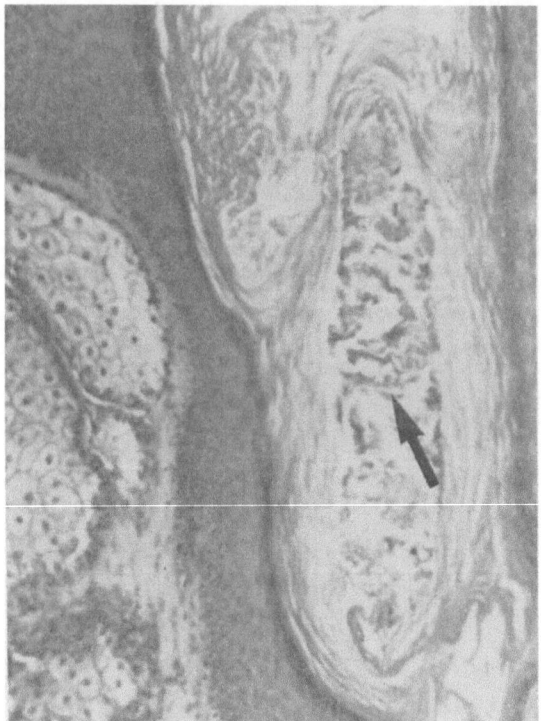

Ill. 8. HE-stained paraffin section. Colonies of propionibacterium acnes in the
follicular content (×160)

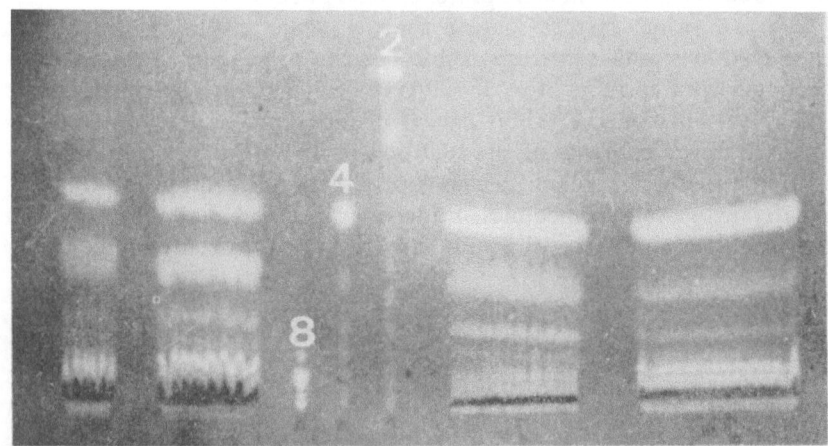

Ill. 9. Thin-layer chromatographic separation of the porphyrins produced by propionibacterium acnes [65]. 2 protoporphyrins; 4 coproporphyrins; 8 uroporphyrins

The lipases were initially thought to be the most important, since they lead to the cleavage of free fatty acids from the triglycerides of the sebum [139, 201, 254], and the amount of free fatty acids—which were regarded as an irritant—is higher in the follicular content of acne patients than in healthy skin. Puhvel and Sakamoto [192], however, have demonstrated experimentally that free fatty acids have a comedogenic and skin-irritating effect only at unphysiologically high concentration.

In addition to this, other enzymes have been described [89, 142] which either metabolize the horny and sebaceous substances to toxin and skin-irritating substances or damage the follicular epithelium itself and thus cause ruptures in the follicular wall. Proteases, for example, attack and destroy the keratin substance, and hyaluronidases decompose the intercellular cement, thereby increasing the permeability of the follicular wall and allowing irritating factors to spread into the surrounding tissue [85].

2. Porphyrin Production

Porphyrins, which have only recently received attention, are metabolic products of *P. acnes*. The presence of porphyrins in the follicle was discovered by means of ostiofollicular red fluorescence of certain skin areas on inspection under Wood light (specially filtered UVA light with maximum emission of 3,600 Å in a darkened room) [14, 161]. This red fluorescence occurs particularly in the centrofacial area, but also in other seborrhoeic areas of skin. A topographic study of 500 subjects by Bues [22] produced the following finding: the nasolabial sulcus luminesced in 54% of the subjects studied, the auricle in 34% and the mentolabial sulcus in 24%. The frequency in seborrhoeic subjects is considerably higher than in non-seborrhoeic subjects.

Inspection of follicular filaments in the fluorescence microscope shows that the fluorescence is bound to amorphous material: keratin masses and lipids are interfused with porphyrins. However, examination of *P. acnes* culture under Wood light confirms that the production of porphyrin is bound to the diphtheroid organism.

Differentiated studies by Formanek *et al.* [65] of individually isolated strains of *P. acnes* using thin-layer chromatography reveal an extremely broad spectrum of porphyrins covering all fractions from 2 to 8 carboxyl groups (Ill. 9).

Since quantity-dependent, erythematous reactions occur after intracutaneous injection of porphyrin extracts and subsequent irradiation with UVA [152, 205], the question arose of whether porphyrins also play a role in the pathogenesis of acne. Comparative studies of pure cultures of *P. acnes* grown from inflammatory acne lesions on the one hand, and from non-inflammatory seborrhoeic follicular filaments on the other revealed for acne patients a generally higher production of porphyrins, a pronounced tendency for porphyrins to

Table 10. *Porphyrin production of propiniobacterium acnes in acne and seborrhoea [by Fanta et al. (57)]*

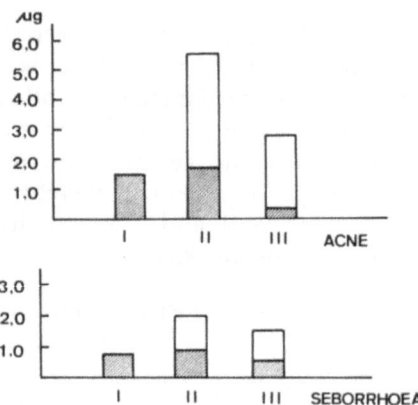

▨ Amount of porphyrins obtained from the bacterial colonies, ▭ amount of porphyrins released into the culture by the colonies (*I–III* three cultures)

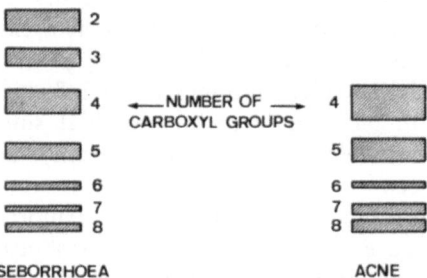

Fig. 5. Schematic representation of thin-layer chromatographic separation of the porphyrins produced by propionibacterium acnes in seborrhoea and acne [by Fanta *et al.* (57)]. (*2–8:* Number of carboxyl groups of the porphyrin fractions)

spread into the surroundings (Table 10), and also a shift in the fractions inasmuch as coproporphyrin appeared as by far the strongest band, whereas protoporphyrins were demonstrated in larger amounts in seborrhoeic patients (Fig. 5).

It might be concluded from these studies that a metabolically more active mutant of *Propionibacterium acnes* is present in acne [57].

3. Antigen Character

The antigen character of *Propionibacterium acnes* has recently also come to be considered significant for the development of inflammatory changes [104]: whereas antibody titers to *Staphylococcus epidermidis* are of approximately the same magnitude in acne patients and healthy controls [191], those to *P. acnes* are present to a marked extent only in patients with inflammatory acne and achieve agglutination titers up to 1 : 40,000 in patients with conglobate acne. Since there are no antibodies in healthy subjects despite *P. acnes* settlement of the skin, the germs apparently develop no antigen character at all in the normal follicle [190]. The titer of antibodies ascribable to IgM class is proportional to the degree of acne.

Antibodies to extracellular antigen components of dialyzed *P. acnes* cultures can also be demonstrated in the serum of acne patients [190].

Whereas the cellular antigens of *P. acnes* lead to skin reactions of the immediate type, the extent of which correlates well with the degree of acne [188], skin reactions of the delayed type to various microbial antigens are reduced in patients with conglobate acne. Since suppression of cellular immunity by *P. acnes* vaccines has been observed in animal experiments, it is assumed that the last-mentioned phenomenon is induced by repeated release of *P. acnes* into the dermis [189].

The responsiveness of the lymphocytes of acne patients to *P. acnes* is increased, whereas that to Phythaemagglutinin (PHA) remains within the normal range [193]. Finally, *P. acnes* stimulation of the reticuloendothelial system (RES) to macrophage production and chemotactic response, to which the accumulation of polymorphonuclear leucocytes in the initial stage of inflammation corresponds, has been demonstrated [1, 34, 84, 221].

Immunofluorescent-optical tests showed C_3 deposits, partly without, partly with a simultaneous deposit of immunoglobulin on the subepithelial membrane of the comedo and the surrounding cell walls. It remains unclear, however, whether the *P. acne* is also responsible for this complementary activation, which, in respect to the cellular immune reaction, represents a very early occurrence in the course of inflammation.

Numerous findings support the presence of a *P. acnes*-induced immunopathological process in severe acne cases. The positive effect of intralesional injections of corticosteroids in nodulocystic acne can be regarded as further confirmation of this.

II. The Forms of Acne

A large group of diseases is placed together under the term "acne" on the basis of the concurrence of pathomechanical, clinical, and histological criteria. The characteristic lesions always develop from follicles in seborrhoeic areas.

The disease is divided into three sub-groups—endogenous acne, exogenous acne, and acneiform eruptions or "drug acne"—according to which additional factors are recognized. Whereas in endogenous acne genetic factors together with the largely physiological and developmental changes occurring at the time of puberty are sufficient for the lesions to become manifest, a predisposition together with additional noxae, e.g. chemical and physical irritants or drugs, must be present for the disease to erupt in its other two forms [123, 171, 198].

A. Endogenous Acne

1. Acne vulgaris

The dominant form in the "endogenous" group is acne vulgaris, or pubertal acne, the manifestations of which are largely restricted to the face, shoulders and V = area of the chest and which is subdivided into comedonal acne (Ill. 10, 11), papulopustular acne (Ill. 12), and a form of acne with persisting nodes and cysts (nodulocystic acne) (Ill. 13) depending on the predominance of individual acne lesions. These variants can, however, overlap. The severity of the disease is graded in degrees according to the number of lesions.

Classification according to Plewig and Kligman [176]:

Comedonal acne

1st degree	less than 10 comedones on one side
2nd degree	10–25 comedones on one side
3rd degree	25–50 comedones on one side
4th degree	more than 50 comedones on one side

Papulopustular acne

1st degree	less than 10 papulopustules on one side
2nd degree	10–20 papulopustules on one side
3rd degree	20–30 papulopustules on one side
4th degree	more than 30 papulopustules on one side

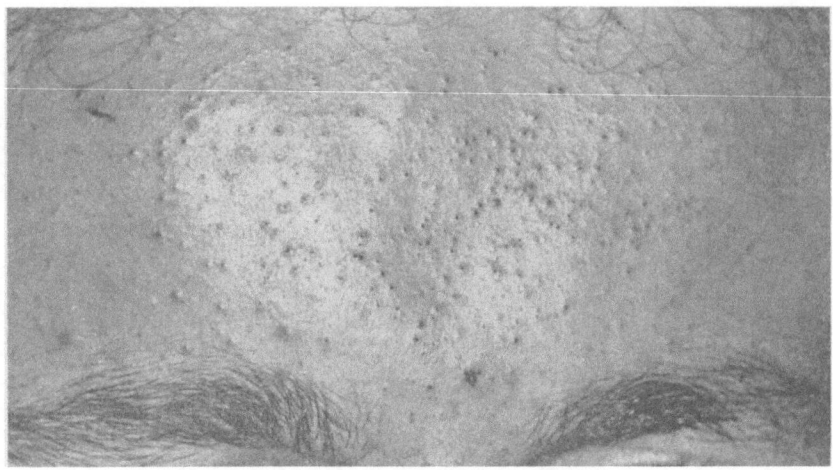

Ill. 10. Comedonal acne: "open" comedones

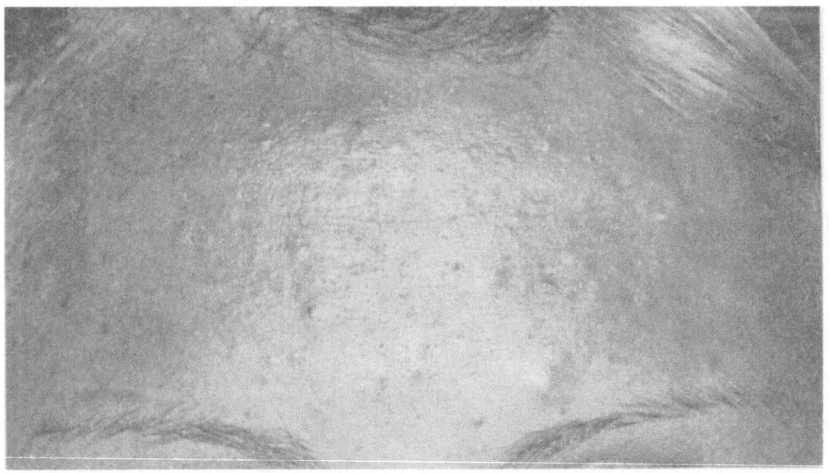

Ill. 11. Comedonal acne: "closed" comedones

Acne with persisting nodes

1st degree	less than 5 nodules on one side
2nd degree	5–10 nodules on one side
3rd degree	10–15 nodules on one side
4th degree	more than 15 nodules on one side

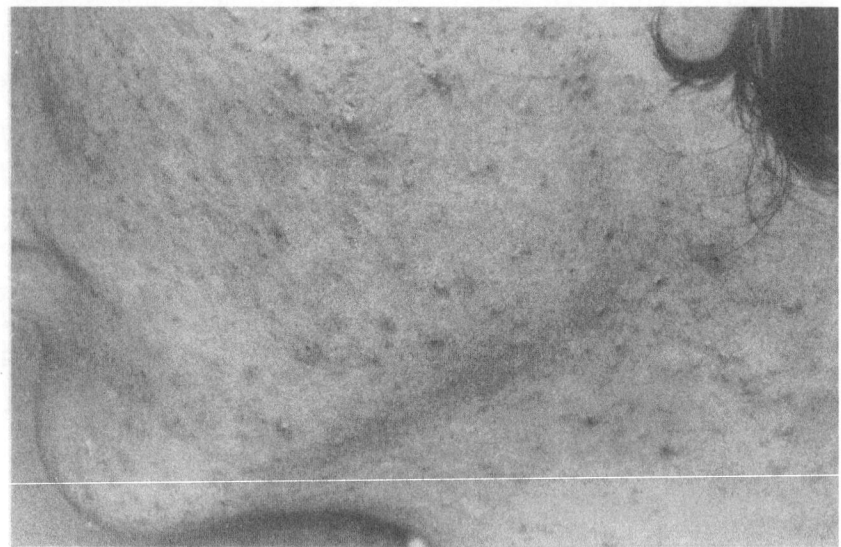

Ill. 12. Papulopustular acne

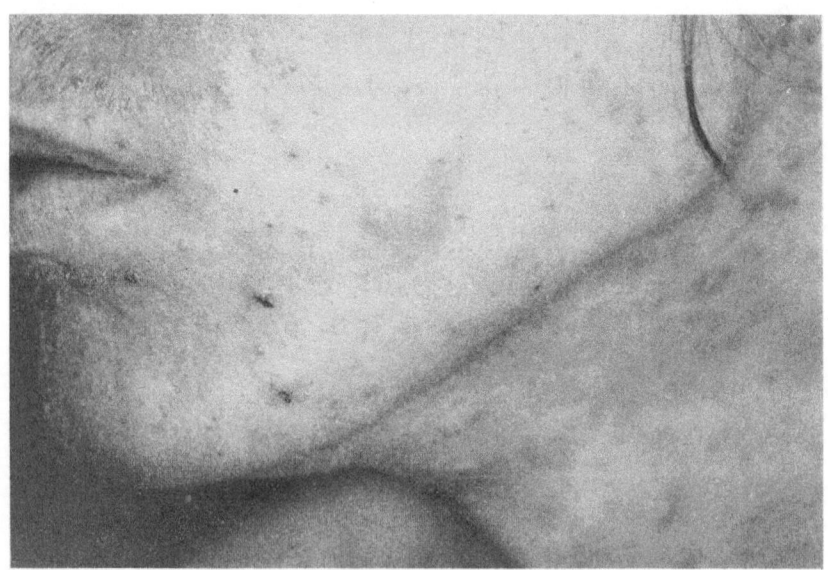

Ill. 13. Nodulocystic acne

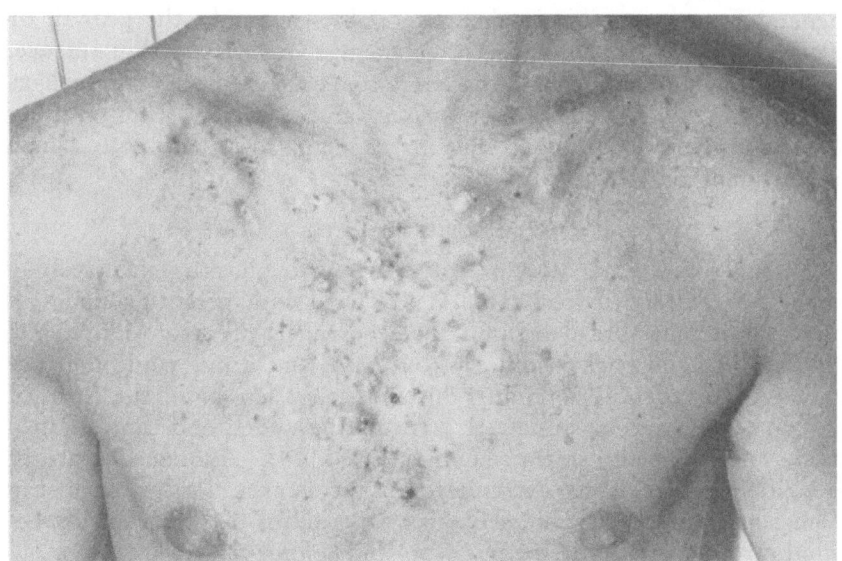

Ill. 14. Conglobate acne

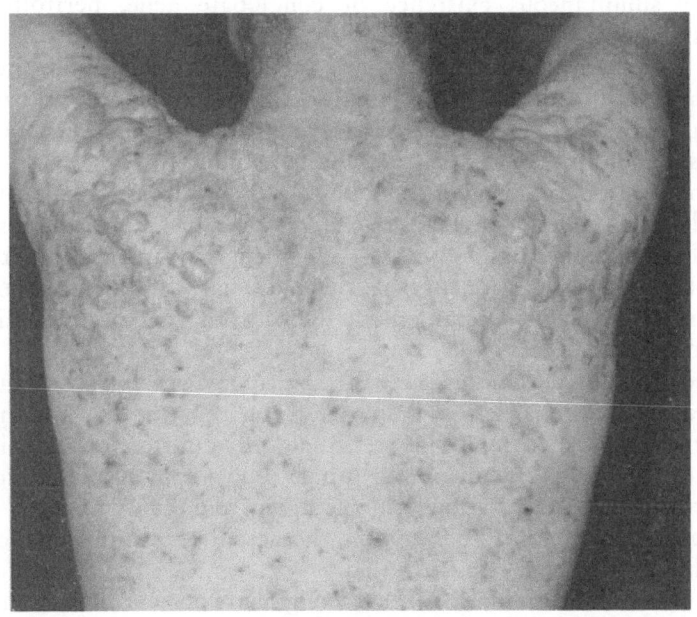

Ill. 15. Keloid acne

Gram-negative folliculitis is a special form of papulopustular acne: long-term antibiotic therapy inhibits not only the growth of *P. acnes* but also that of the other commensals of the skin surface, and can as a result lead to proliferation of resistant germs such as *Klebsiella, Enterobacter, Salmonellae,* and *Proteus.* The resulting folliculitis can be controlled only by changing to an antibiotic whose spectrum of action also covers gram-negative germs.

2. Conglobate Acne

Conglobate acne affects primarily—through not exclusively—male patients and differs from severe acne with persisting nodes in that the lesions spread beyond the seborrhoeic areas of skin to the entire chest and back, shoulders, buttocks, and arms, while the face is less involved [217]. Highly inflammatory lesions in the form of colliquative necrosis, colliquative fistulating nodes, and canal-shaped undermining of the skin predominate (Ill. 14). Another feature of conglobate acne is its extremely chronic course: fresh lesions can sometimes appear continuously over a period of decades, leaving behind atrophic and hypertrophic scars and keloids (Ill. 15).

Plewig and Kligman [176] have subdivided this form according to the number of areas affected: the term "acne triade" was coined for the simultaneous existence of conglobate acne, perifolliculitis capitis abscedens et suffodiens, and hidranenitis suppurativa axillaris, while "acne tetrade" is present when the inguinal apocrine glands are also involved. Finally, "acne pentade" also includes the presence of undermining abscesses in the perianal and sacral region, and pilonidal sinuses (synonym: "dermatitis perianalis fistulosa").

An additional male gonosome has occasionally been demonstrated in males with severe conglobate acne, and this has led to the assumption that the acne in these cases—so-called XYY-acne—might be a phenotypic manifestation of the chromosomal aberration [176]. A similar phenomenon is assumed for the cases of acne occurring in the Down's syndrome.

Because of the importance of additional precipitating factors, tropical acne is regarded as a special form, representing a transition to the exogenous forms of acne. Renewed eruption of acne in the form of conglobate acne on the upper body can occur in tropical climates in male patients beyond the age of puberty who have a history of acne; attempts to pinpoint the actual precipitating factor—heat, humidity?—have so far failed.

A grave and fulminant form of conglobate acne is acne fulminans, which has so far only been observed in males and the symptoms of which have been described by Kelly and Burns [117]:

Acute onset

Picture of conglobate acne with ulcerations

Generally toxic symptoms with high fever, polyarthralgia, increased blood sedimentation rate, lytic bone lesions [164] and leukaemic blood changes

Therapy-resistant to antibiotics, but responds relatively quickly to corticosteroids.

Because of its clinical course this variant was initially regarded as a kind of Schwartzman phenomenon or Arthus's reaction. However, apart from its therapeutic responsiveness to corticosteroids, other findings suggest that—as is also generally assumed in conglobate acne—immunological factors play a special role in this disease [196, 248]: skin reactions to viral and bacterial antigens are reduced in patients with acne fulminans, while an IgE increase can be observed in the humoral defence [230]. Thus, increased humoral immunity with simultaneously decreased cell-mediated immunity is probably present.

3. Acne with Particular Involvement of Hormonal Factors

Although androgenic stimulation of the sebaceous glands or increased androgen metabolism of the skin is a prerequisite for the start of the pathological process in all acne variants, some special forms stand out by virtue of a particularly pronounced dependence on hormones, characterized by endogenously or exogenously induced hormonal fluctuations.

The first of these from a chronological point of view is neonatal acne (Fig. 16), which develops in the first week of life and lasts only about 2 months [47]. After this period it usually heals up spontaneously. The primarily inflammatory, follicular eruptions are strictly limited to the face and appear in groups on the forehead and cheeks. A family disposition is a frequent observation. The prerequisite of an adequate production of sebum for the development of the acne lesions is present here as well: the skin surface lipids increase greatly in the first week of life; although the values display great individual variations, they average about the same magnitude as in adults. The production of sebum ceases almost completely by the sixth month of life following a gradual decrease.

This initial activity of the sebaceous glands is related to the pathogenesis of mammary gland swelling and vaginal bleeding in neonates and is attributed to general stimulation of steroid production after birth [214]. While the plasma levels of cortisone and adrenal testosterone decrease in girls after the first week of life, testosterone remains elevated for 2–3 months in boys and does not decrease to the pre-adrenarche values until after approximately 7 months: a negative

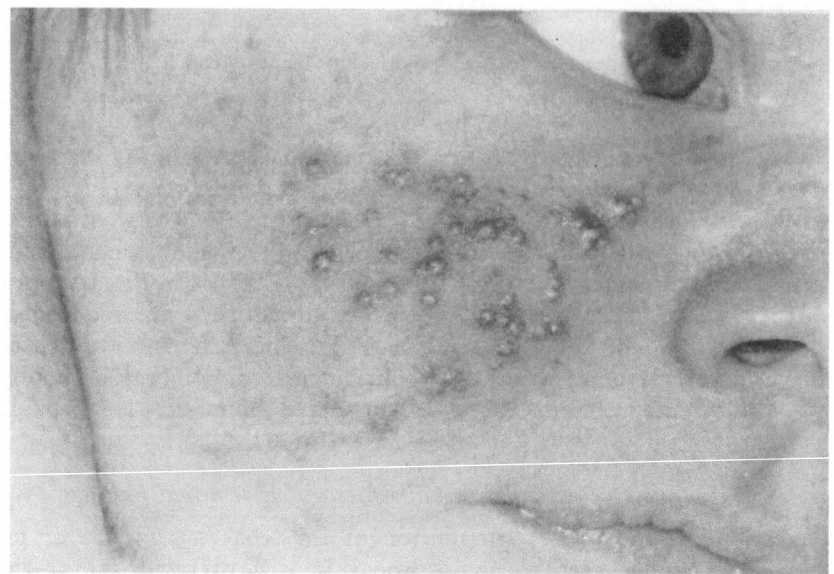

Ill. 16. Neonatal acne

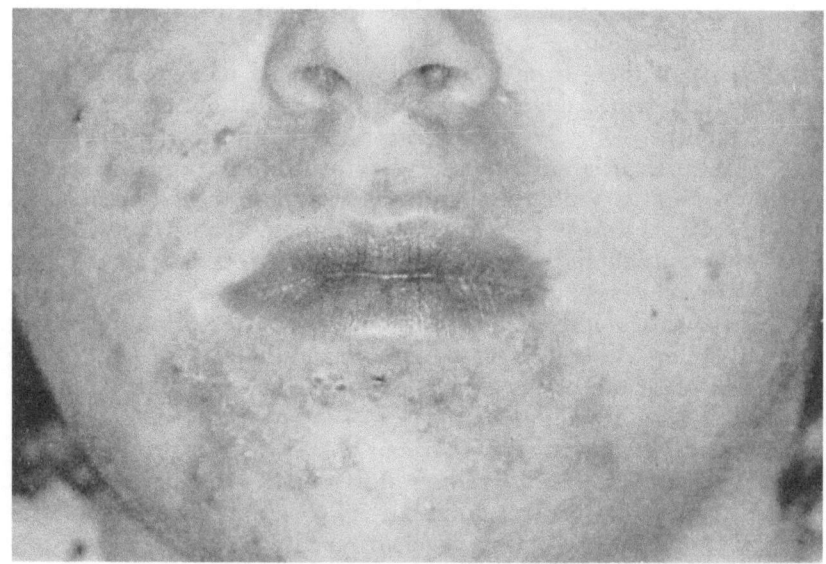

Ill. 17. Postpubertal progestational acne (29-year-old female patient)

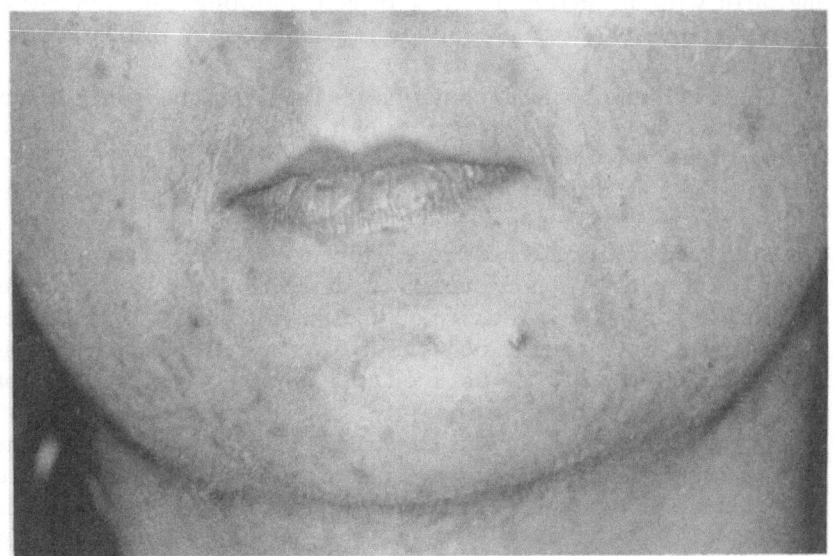

Ill. 18. Acne with signs of androgenization

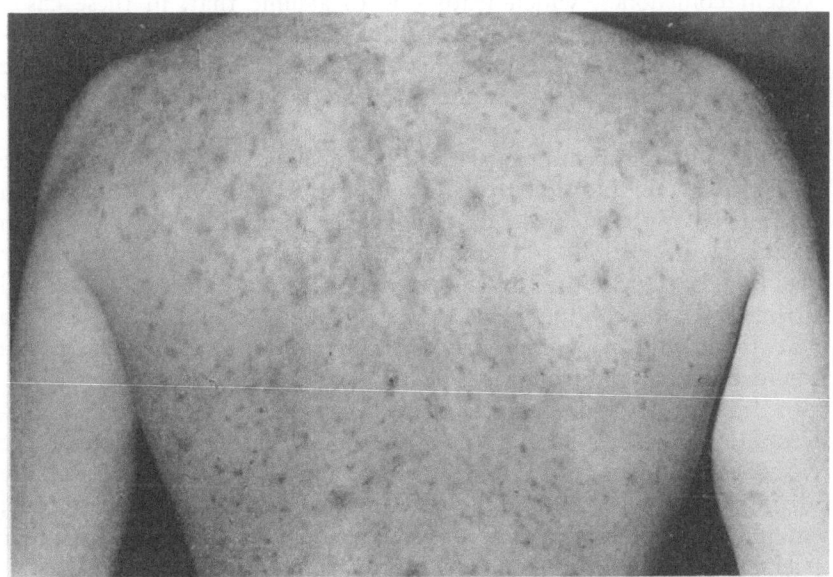

Ill. 19. Acne on the back of an adult male (30-year-old patient)

feed-back mechanism induced by the rapid fall of oestrogens following birth with an increased release of gonadotropins and stimulation
of testicular testosterone production is assumed to be responsible for
this process [64].

This could also be the explanation for infantile acne, which occurs
primarily in boys from the third month of life and which develops
in the presence of a particular genetic sensitivity of the sebaceous
glands—there is usually a family disposition to infantile acne as
well—and this could be viewed as a reaction to these somewhat higher
but still physiological testosterone values. The fact that no other
signs of androgenization are observed at the same time is an indication of the particular sensitivity of the skin receptors. If comedones
predominate, however, the possible involvement of external precipitating factors—the use of head oil and ointment—in the sense of
acne venenata must be considered [15].

Premenstrual acne cannot be strictly distinguished from acne
vulgaris of the female in general, since existing acne deteriorates to
some extent in the premenstrual period in almost 80% of female
patients [158]. Occasionally, however, the sudden appearance of
painful, inflammatory nodes in the region of the chin and lateral
cheeks represents the only manifestation of acne. There are no pre-
existent comedones, which leads one to assume that, in these cases,
rupture and inflammation of the follicular wall occur without preceding disturbed hornification in the follicular epithelium. At the same
time these patients report sudden, marked greasiness of the hair, or
distinct effluvium.

The sudden appearance of these premenstrual acne lesions can be
explained by the physiological hormonal fluctuations which occur in
the normal biphasic cycle of the female [75]: oestrogens—and in
particular oestradiol—fall sharply after a maximum preovulatory
level one day before the LH (luteotropic hormone) peak and then fall
further after a second increase in the luteal phase. Following a steep
increase at mid-cycle, the progesterone level remains high in the
second phase of the cycle (Table 11). Lastly, attention has recently
been drawn to a slight increase of testosterone and dehydroepiandrosterone at mid-cycle [163]. Increased androgenic stimulation of the
sebaceous glands results from the interaction of these factors: the
fall in the oestrogen levels, the plateau-like increase of progesterone,
which can possibly be metabolized to androgen in the skin under
special conditions, and the increase in ovarian androgens.

The androgenic partial effect of progestogens plays a major role
in postpubertal progestational acne in particular [20]: this form of
acne occurs in females with a history of transient pubertal acne from

the mid-twenties onwards and displays mainly papulopustular lesions and persisting nodes in the region of the nasolabial folds and chin (Ill. 17). Another feature of this type of acne is pronounced premenstrual exacerbation. The condition deteriorates dramatically under the use of oral contraceptives with a progestogen of the 19-nortestosterone class. A striking feature is its resistance to antibiotics

Table 11. *Serum levels of 17-β-oestradiol and progesterone during a spontaneous ovulatory cycle [by Gitsch et al. (75)]. (Day "0" is the day of the cycle on which the LH peak occurs)*

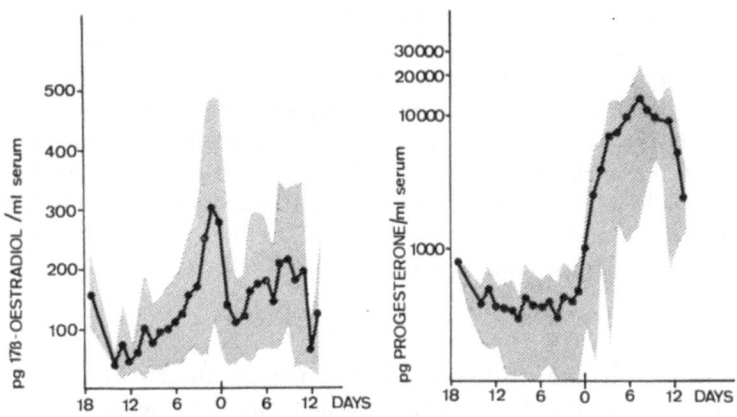

and the various topical measures, and its rapid response to an ovulation inhibitor containing a progestational component with an antiandrogenic action.

Androgenetic acne [144] of the adult female—a highly inflammatory condition—can be interpreted as a symptom of overproduction of ovarian or adrenal androgens in the presence of ovarian tumours, *e.g.* the Stein-Leventhal syndrome, luteomas, and adrenocortical tumours. The additional increased production of hydrocortisone can further exacerbate the course of the disease in the form of steroid acne. Other signs of virilization, *e.g.* hirsutism and androgenic effluvium, are usually also present in this condition (Ill. 18). Acne on the back of the adult male (Ill. 19) should, perhaps, also be placed in this group of hormonedependent forms of acne. There is usually no history of acne, but follicular papules appear after puberty and up to about the age of 50. The papules are relatively resistant to therapy and, as in premenstrual acne, the preceding stage of comedones is absent.

B. Exogenous Acne

In addition to the obligatory pathogenic factors, external influences come to bear in the group of exogenous forms of acne.

1. Acne venenata

The chemical substances which provoke acne venenata are primarily organic hydrocarbon compounds and lipids: a comedogenic effect has been demonstrated, for example, for numerous cosmetics in experiments on the rabbit ear [71]. On long-term use and in the presence of an acne disposition, these preparations lead to the development of numerous closed comedones the picture of cosmetic acne [112] (Ill. 20). Scalp oil-provoked pomatum acne and detergent acne [147] following too frequent and too intensive washing with comedogenic detergents fall into this category. Oil acne and tar and pitch acne are occupational diseases which develop relatively quickly after contact with these substances, the picture being dominated by open comedones (Ill. 21). Most frequently affected are mechanics, ship builders, and road workers. The mechanical friction of oil-saturated clothing promotes inflammatory lesions.

2. Chloracne

Chlorine in the form of chlorinated aromatic hydrocarbons, such as those reduced as waste products in the chemical industry during the manufacture of herbicides and insecticides, e.g. in the form of tetrachlordibenz-p-dioxin (TCDD), provoke chloracne via skin contact and inhalation. The changes in the skin are then the first symptom of poisoning caused by this carcinogenic, mutagenic and teratogenic substance. The development of this disease is usually acute and sometimes epidemic; a polymorphous, severe condition of comedonal acne with general signs of intoxication develops. The course is extremely prolonged because the chemically very stable, highly toxic substances remain in the organism for a long time. There is no known antidote at the present time.

3. Physical Acne

Senile comedones provoked by actinic irritation—in the full picture of Favre-Racouchot's disease—and the comedones appearing after X-ray therapy are not quite correctly regarded as belonging to the group of exogenous forms of acne.

Comedones following X-ray therapy, however, result simply from activation of the proliferative activity in the follicular epithelium by

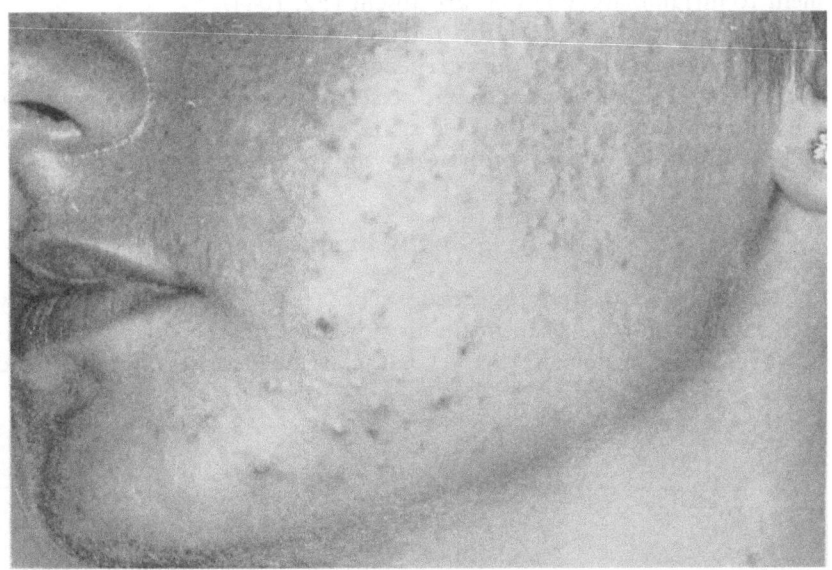

Ill. 20. Cosmetic acne

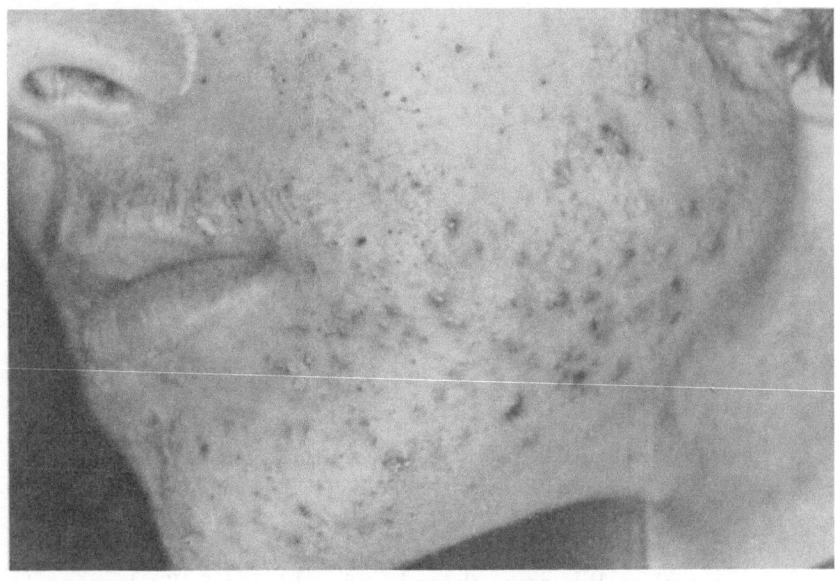

Ill. 21. Oil acne (mechanic)

the rays: ruptures in the follicular epithelium and further development to inflammatory lesions are absent [52, 108].

Attempts to classify Majorca acne have so far failed: small follicular nodules develop on the forehead and temples, upper body, and upper arms in people holidaying at seaside resorts. It is not known whether the inducing factors are again actinic stimuli or whether the use of suntan oils or contamination by oily seawater is responsible.

C. Acneiform Eruptions

Acneiform eruptions or "drug acne" [20] are a comparatively rare side effect which can occur in systemic and topical use of various drugs and chemicals [96]. Characteristic features are the rapid

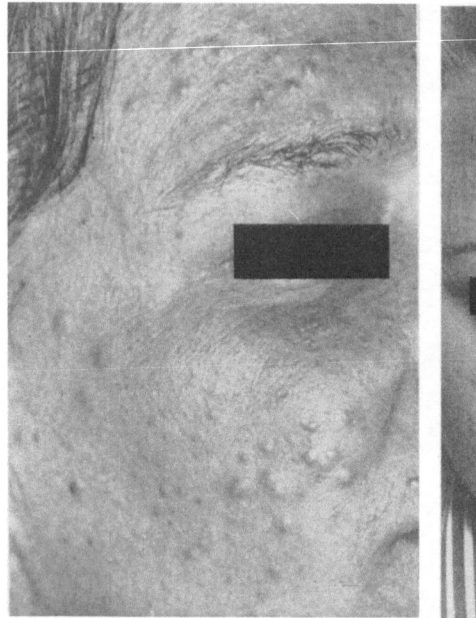 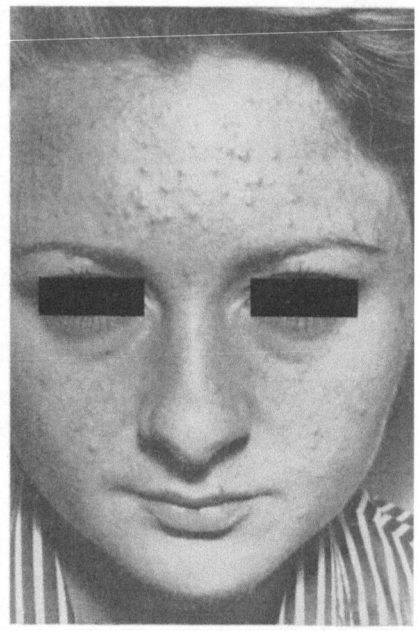

Ill. 22   Ill. 23

Ill. 22. Drug-induced acneform eruptions (after iodinated preparation)
Ill. 23. Drug-induced acneiform eruptions (after vitamin B complex)

development of the lesions and the monomorphous clinical picture with its smooth, solid, dome-shaped and reddened follicular papules which appear mainly in the typical acne areas. Comedones are not usually observed until considerably later, and there are no cysts. The main group of people affected are patients beyond the age of puberty with a history of acne; the acneiform eruptions can, however, also develop to aggravate existing acne.

The main inducing agents are reported to be iodide (Ill. 22) [97], bromide, isonicotinic acid hydrazide [31] vitamins B 6 and B 12 [20] (Ill. 23), sedative and antiepileptics, tetracyclines, ACTH [223], and glucocorticoids [174]. Acneiform eruptions have recently also been observed under photochemotherapy [99]. The causal association with the drug can be confirmed by reproduction of the lesions after re-exposure.

Apart from ACTH, which is by far the most frequent inducer of acneiform eruptions and which has a stimulatory effect on the sebaceous glands in animal experiments comparable to that of tes-tosterone [93, 233], none of the other substances mentioned has a sebotropic effect. In particular, no increase of sebum production has been observed on systemic or topical administration of glucocorticoids either in animal experiments or in man [208, 140]. On the contrary, glucocorticoids have been said to support the sebaceous gland-in-hibitory effect of oestrogens in patients with the adrenogenital syn-drome [181].

A comedogenic property of the drugs mentioned can also be ruled out.

The histological picture of steroid acne with circumscribed spongi-osis and necrosis in the follicular epithelium suggests primary damage to the follicular wall with the subsequent development of intra- and perifollicular abscesses [109, 174].

III. Therapy of Acne

The factors of the pathomechanisms of acne so far known dictate that the desired effects of therapy should be antiseborrhoeic, comedolytic, and bacteriostatic. Immunological acne therapy must still be regarded as being in its infancy.

In view of the variability of the disease, however, it would be unrealistic to expect satisfactory therapeutic results from just one method of treatment—combined therapy with a shifting point of emphasis should be given preference. If possible, the most suitable form of therapy is chosen on the one hand according to aetiological aspects—*e.g.* elimination of external factors—and, on the other, according to the clinical picture depending on the predominance of individual acne lesions. The respective degree of severity of the various forms of acne is also of paramount importance.

The following is a review—supplemented by personal findings—of recent therapeutic developments which have become established in the treatment of acne over the last few years.

A. Topical Therapy

1. Retinoic Acid

Therapy with topically applied retinoic acid—an all-*trans* retinal—has been shown to be far superior to the keratolytic substances—*e.g.* salicylic acid, sulphur, resorcin, beta naphthol—previously used in the treatment of acne [273]. While other desquamative agents lead to relaxation and thickening of the horny layer via lysis of the intercellular substance, retinoic acid causes stimulation of the normal mitotic activity of keratinizing epithelia and, at the same time, inhibition of keratin production, thus leading to parakeratosis and thinning of the horny layer [121, 272]. Keratinocyte proliferation is also increased in the infundibulum of the follicle [220, 244]. The coherence of the horny lamellae is consequently dissolved and the keratin plug thus lifted out of the follicular infundibulum. Genuine comedolysis takes place. In addition, concomitant hyperaemization allows better removal of toxins and, on combined systemic antibiotic therapy, an increased local concentration of the antibiotics.

Erythema, oedema and scaling occur at the start of therapy, and the patient may complain of itching and smarting. Increased transformation of comedones into papular and pustular lesions usually results in the initial stage from inflammatory concomitant reactions and leucocyte invasion. However, the lesions regress again after a few weeks of continued therapy, a process which can be helped considerably by combining the retinoic acid treatment with antibiotics or benzoyl peroxide. The skin becomes rosy and shiny after about 8 weeks of therapy.

0.05% formulations are used, lotion or gel being chosen for severe seborrhoea and the cream for less greasy skin. Treatment should be initiated with one application per day, particularly in lightly pigmented patients, and the dosage increased to two applications per day after the first pustular eruption; the start of treatment should be more intensive in the case of patients with darker pigmentation. The therapy should be continued at the same intensity until the desired effect is achieved—after about 10–12 weeks—after which the dosage should be reduced to two applications per week as maintenance therapy.

Because of the increased sensitivity of the skin, the simultaneous use of substances with a marked irritant action, examples of which are still used in acne therapy, should be avoided and the skin cleansed as gently as possible; exposure to sunlight should also be avoided. Regular office visits and the psychological management of the patient are important—particularly at the start of treatment—to ensure that the therapy is carried out consistently during the phase of deterioration as well.

2. Benzoyl Peroxide (BP)

Clinical trials of benzoyl peroxide-containing preparations reveal above all a rapid response of inflammatory acne lesions, while existing comedones respond only slowly [53, 143, 167, 252].

The current conception about the mechanism of action of BP is based on the one hand on the observation of a decrease of microbial settlement after 14 days' use of a 10% formulation, similar to that under systemic tetracycline administration [72], and, on the other, on the demonstration of a significant decrease of the percentage of free fatty acids in the skin surface lipids, which are regarded as a parameter for the presence of propionibacterium acnes [79]. It was concluded from this that BP has a primarily bacteriostatic effect which—as with various other peroxides [199]—is probably based on the conversion of bacterial amino acids to panthothionic acid. However, the gel base which is usually used, which is composed of colloidal magnesium-aluminium silicate, hydroxyethylene lauryl ether, citric acid, absolute ethanol, and distilled water, and which has been found to be the best for topical use, appears to play an essential role in the reduction of the microbial settlement [50].

Marked desquamation and regression of the oily aspect of acne

skin can also be observed under topical treatment with BP [53]. It
has been assumed in this connection that, as with salicylic acid, the
benzoic acid which arises on contact of BP with organic substances
exerts a keratolytic effect via lysis of the intercellular substance and
the resultant relaxation of the epidermis leads to the dry appearance
of the skin [72]. Pertinent studies using autoradiography produced
interesting results after 3 weeks' topical use of a 5% formulation:

Table 12. *Labelling indices in the epidermis, follicular infundibulum and sebaceous
glands before* ☐ *and after* ▨ *treatment with benzoyl peroxide [by
Fanta (58)]*

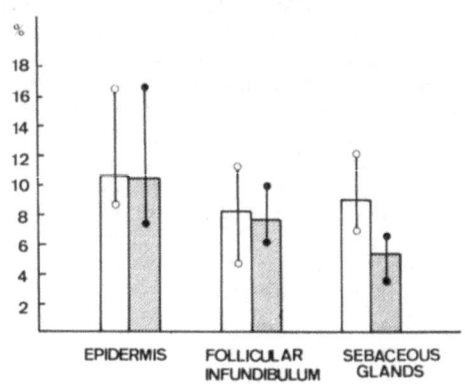

Statistical calculation using the t-test:

Sebaceous glands:	☐	▨	
x̄	9.11	5.55	
σ	2.1	1.4	p > 0.0001

although the labelling index remained the same in the epidermis and
follicular infundibulum, it decreased significantly in the germinal
cells of the sebaceous glands [58] (Table 12). These findings have
been confirmed by further examinations of the cell kinetics by determination of the mitotic index and the length of the S-phase and
in addition by histoplanimetric studies [80]. Findings from quantitative
determination of skin surface lipids agreed with this: both the casual
level and the replacement sum decreased significantly after 4 weeks'
treatment [56] (Table 13). In agreement with other authors, this
study series also revealed a shift of the individual lipid fractions, the
reduction of free fatty acids appearing to be the most important.
The simultaneous reduction of the triglycerides too points to the re-
tardation of the sebaceous gland development through the use of
benzoyl peroxide.

Thus, in addition to its bacteriostatic and desquamative properties, benzoyl peroxide would also appear to have a sebostatic effect, the mechanism of which is still unclarified.

Benzoyl peroxide in a 5 or 10% formulation is applied once daily to the affected areas of skin. The use can be reduced after about 8 weeks. If excessive scaling occurs, it is advisable to apply an indifferent cooling ointment now and then. A disadvantage is the marked sensitizing potency of BP, which leads to the development of contact eczema in 3–5% of cases.

Table 13. *Skin surface lipid values before* ⬜ *and after* ▨ *therapy with benzoyl peroxide [by Fanta (56)]*

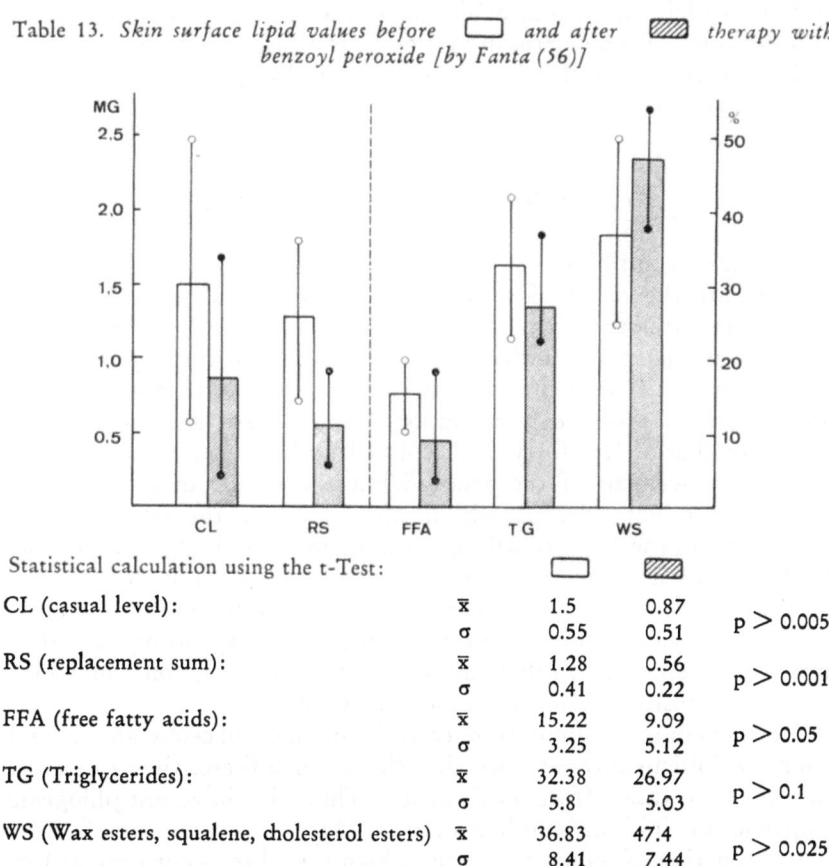

Statistical calculation using the t-Test:

		⬜	▨	
CL (casual level):	x̄	1.5	0.87	p > 0.005
	σ	0.55	0.51	
RS (replacement sum):	x̄	1.28	0.56	p > 0.001
	σ	0.41	0.22	
FFA (free fatty acids):	x̄	15.22	9.09	p > 0.05
	σ	3.25	5.12	
TG (Triglycerides):	x̄	32.38	26.97	p > 0.1
	σ	5.8	5.03	
WS (Wax esters, squalene, cholesterol esters)	x̄	36.83	47.4	p > 0.025
	σ	8.41	7.44	

3. Topical Antibiotic Therapy

The golden rule of topical antibiotic therapy should be that only those drugs are chosen which cause the least sensitization [63]. Although tetracyclines—*e.g.* tetracycline hydrochloride in a 5% formu-

lation with DMSO [78]—exert a favourable influence on the course
of acne, they do not fulfill this condition; topically applied erythromycin, on the other hand, has so far caused no sensitization. Good
results have been achieved with the fat-soluble erythromycin derivatives (erythromycin base, propionate and stearate) in 2% formulations [63, 71, 148].

The use of clindamycin phosphate, which should not be applied
over too large a surface on account of the danger of colitis after high
absorption [12, 202, 223], brings some success, according to some
authors, which equals that achieved by the systematic administration
of antibiotics. Problematic, however, in the case of all the substances
so far mentioned, is the production of a stable preparation suitable
for an acne skin.

B. Systemic Antibiotic Treatment

The use of antibiotics was based essentially on the idea that acne
pustules are the result of secondary infection. The maintenance of
this theory after the observation that only *P. acnes* is of major importance in the pathomechanism is based on the observations that
P. acnes is sensitive to broad-band antibiotics *in vitro* and that oral
administration leads to a reduction of *P. acnes*—as demonstrated
by the number of free fatty acids split off, which is also accompanied
by an improvement of the acne. While the results under penicillin
and sulfonamides were usually disappointing or the percentage of
side effects in the form of allergic exanthem is too high, tetracyclines
proved to be a rational, effective, and relatively safe drug. They
have been well tested for 30 years in respect of toxicity and tolerance,
and for this reason alone—with the exception of erythromycin—they
should be preferred to other, more recent antibiotics, some of which
also have a positive influence on acne vulgaris.

Tetracyclines accumulate selectively in the sebaceous glands and
enter the follicular canal with the sebum; once there, they can exert
their bacteriostatic effect on *P. acnes*. They also have antiphlogistic
properties via inhibition of leucotaxis [175].

A reduction of sebum synthesis, which is said to occur even at low
dosage, has also been suggested on the basis of clinical observations
of therapeutic success in seborrhoea. The inhibition of microbial
lipases demonstrated *in vitro* probably plays only a minor role *in
vivo*. The administration of oxytetracycline hydrochloride, tetracycline hydrochloride or tetracycline-L-methylenelysin is to be recommended, since these preparations lead to gastric complaints and

diarrhoea to a much lesser extent than, for example, dimethyl chlortetracycline and chlortetracycline. The synthetic derivative methacycline, which was created by dehydration of oxytetracycline, has
recently also proved to be extremely effective, and even superior to
other tetracyclines; this high efficacy makes it possible—as with
tetracycline-L-methylenelysin—to reduce the average daily dose of
1.0 g required with other tetracyclines to 0.6 g [49].

Allergic reactions and photodermatoses usually only occur after
dimethyl chlortetracycline, but all patients under tetracycline treatment should be given a general warning about exposure to intensive
sunlight. Serious damage, e.g. to liver and kidneys, is unlikely under
the dosage employed [9], but disturbed liver and renal function
should nevertheless be ruled out before the start of treatment [32].
Tetracycline medication is contraindicated in pregnancy: the child's
teeth might later turn yellow and the bone marrow might be disturbed. As with any long-term antibiotic therapy, a watch should be
kept for the increased occurrence of mycoses, e.g. blastomyces colpitis.

The macrolide derivative erythromycin mentioned above has also
proved its suitability for acne therapy, and displays the lowest side
effects rate [279]. Lincomycin and clindamycin—likewise effective
anti-acne agents—should not be used because of possible complica-
tions in the form of pseudomembranous colitis [223].

The initial dosage should not exceed 1,000 mg tetracycline hydrochloride or
600 mg tetracycline-L-methylenelysin or methacycline per day. As soon as clinical
improvement becomes apparent—after 2–4 weeks—the dosage can be reduced to
a maintenance level of 250 mg and 150 mg, respectively.

Since the maximum absorption value is 250 mg, the initial dose should be distributed throughout the day. The tablets are best taken with a lot of liquid, although milk should be avoided because of the great binding capacity of tetracyclines to calcium. Absorption of tetracyclines is incomplete and subject to great
individual variations, which could be a reason for therapeutic failures.

An initial dose of 1,000 mg followed a few weeks later by a maintenance dose
of 250 mg is also recommended for erythromycin.

The treatment of acne vulgaris with antibiotics, which is indicated
above all in papulopustular forms of acne and conglobate acne, is a
long-term proposal which must be continued for many months until
a switch can be made to topical therapy alone. Concurrent desquamative treatment, e.g. with vitamin A acid, should always be performed because, firstly, existing comedones are not affected by antibiotics and, secondly, local irritation such as that which occurs under
desquamative treatment leads to a higher antibiotic level in the
skin.

C. Hormonal Therapy of Acne

Knowledge about the regulation of sebaceous gland activity by sex hormones has prompted diverse attempts at therapy via influencing this mechanism, the object being to reduce sebum production, *i.e.* to inhibit the effect of androgens on the sebaceous glands. Some of the methods so far proposed look promising:

Firstly, the central effect of oestrogens can bring about reduced androgen production via inhibition of gonadotropin secretion. Over and above this, however, oestrogens also appear to have a direct point of attack at the level of the sebaceous glands, although the mechanism has not yet been clarified [107].

Lastly, they exert an antiphlogistic effect by stimulating the adrenal cortex to secrete cortisone [149].

An earlier opinion expressed in some quarters to the effect that therapeutic success with oestrogens generally can only be achieved at doses associated with a high percentage of side effects—those quoted are metrorrhagia, menorrhagia, Candida colpitis, chloasma, thrombosis and embolism, porphyria cutanea tarda and weight increase due to protein, salt, and water retention—must be refluted: the responsiveness of the sebaceous glands to hormonal influences displays pronounced individual fluctuations, which means that satisfactory therapeutic results can in some cases be achieved with very low doses, *e.g.* 20 mg ethinyl oestradiol. At the same time, it cannot be denied that therapeutic failures have occasionally been observed under a daily dose of 100 µg.

Another way of suppressing androgen-induced stimulation of the sebaceous glands is to use what are known as antiandrogens. These are substances which prevent androgens from exerting their specific activity at the target organs. Since they attack at the level of the target organ itself, they abolish the effect of both endogenous and exogenous androgens.

Many such antiandrogens—both steroids and nonsteroids—are known [266], but very few of them have so far been tested in the treatment of acne.

One of the major points of attack of antiandrogens is inhibition of the 5-α-reductase and, hence, suppression of the metabolism of testosterone to DHT (Fig. 6). The similarity of their chemical structure to that of testosterone makes various steroid hormones in particular suitable for competitive binding of the enzyme. The most potent of these are progesterone [253, 69], androstenedione and deoxycorticosterone [253]. However, none of these substances fulfils the demands made of an antiandrogen for therapeutic use: the chosen substance should itself have no disturbing hormonal activity and should not be a potent precursor of other steroid hormones. Progesterone itself is a precursor in the biosynthesis of androgens, adrostenedione can be further converted to testosterone and thus likewise exert an androgenic effect, while deoxycorticosterone is unsuitable as a therapeutic agent because of its pronounced effect on the mineral balance.

An inhibitor of the 5-α-reductase which appears to fulfil the requirements is 4-androstene-3-one-17-β-carboxylic acid [103], or "17-βc", which is a degradation product of deoxycorticosterone which

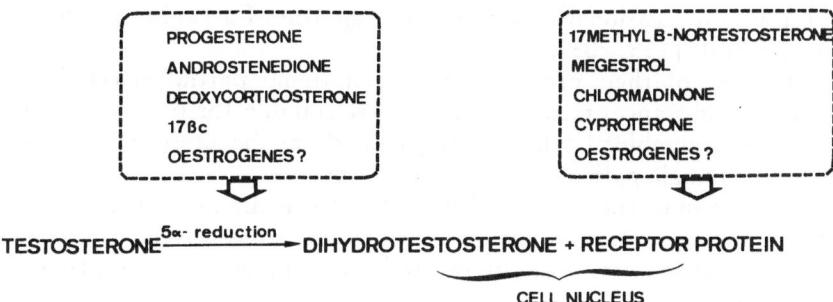

Fig. 6. Possible points of attack for the blockade of androgen metabolism of the skin

displays a pronounced antiandrogenic effect with no central hormonal effect on the flank organ of the hamster, an androgensensitive organ, and which might possibly become an important substance in acne therapy if researched further.

Another point of attack is prevention of DHT binding to the specific receptor protein cytosol prior to transport into the cell nucleus.

17-methyl-B-nortestosterone, a synthetic steroid with a chemical structure similar to that of testosterone and for which competitive inhibition of the receptor protein is assumed, has been described in the American literature [184]. A distinct regression of sebum secretion has been observed both in animals and patients on oral and topical administration [154, 225, 277], although a reduction of the testosterone level under both forms of administration suggests a not insignificant central effect [240] which is corroborated by the occurrence of gynaecomastia in 12 out of 13 treated male patients [29].

The synthetic progesterone derivatives chlormadinone, megestrol, and cyproterone, the antiandrogenic property of which is particularly pronounced in their acetate form, likewise exert their effect via competitive inhibition of the receptor protein. However, these substances cannot be used as anti-acne agents in male patients because of their pronounced effect on other androgen-dependent organs as well-cyproterone acetate, for example, is employed therapeutically at higher dosage in men to suppress drive in sexual deviations and hypersexuality. It was during the investigation of this substance that a distinct regression of sebum production was observed as a concomitant effect [26].

Studies conducted in gestating rats and rabbits after administration of high doses of cyproterone acetate also revealed feminization of male foetuses in the form of a lack of differentiation of male genitals and occasionally even the development of a vagina and mammary glands [155, 203].

Because of their pronounced progestational partial effect, however, the substances mentioned above are suitable for oral contraception when combined with oestrogens and can be prescribed in this form for female patients as acne medication.

Of the numerous forms of hormonal acne therapy so far tested, the most important are discussed and compared in the following chapter, the reports in the literature being supplemented by personal experience.

A fundamental consideration as regards the various forms of hormonal acne therapy is that, although the intervention in the complicated hormone system can be regarded as biological, it is not at all physiological and demands strict selection of the patients. With the possible exception of "17-βc", a purely peripheral therapeutic effect with no central side effect is still not attainable, which is why hormone therapy remains restricted mainly to female patients. If only for psychological reasons and in view of the possible side effects —disturbed spermatogenesis, gynaecomastia—this form of therapy will hardly establish itself for male patients, although amazing results can sometimes be achieved with low doses of oestrogen in men with severe conglobate acne.

It must also be borne in mind that most acne patients are juveniles: current opinion in this respect is that hormone therapy should not be prescribed before the age of 15 in view of epiphyseal closure [10], or not until two years after the menarche in view of normal sexual maturity.

In addition, the guidelines generally valid for the prescription of an oral contraceptive and summarized in the following must also be observed for hormone therapy of acne, isolated administration of oestrogens, and the administration of oestrogens in the form of oral contraceptives [250].

Guidelines for the prescription of oral contraceptives:

Before the start of treatment

>exclusion of contraindications by careful registration of the case history and a general medical examination
>palpatory examination of the genitalia with speculum examination of the cervix and cytological smear control
>palpation of the breasts
>urine check for sugar
>blood pressure measurement

During treatment

at intervals of 6 months

>palpatory examination of the genitalia with speculum examination of the portio
>palpation of the breasts
>urine check for sugar
>blood pressure check

at intervals of 12 months

>cytological smear control
>liver function test in suspected liver damage

The contraindications are:

>a history of thromboembolism during pregnancy
>sickle cell anaemia
>hormone-dependent malignant tumours
>pregnancy
>existing hepatocyte damage
>acute liver infections
>a history of jaundice of pregnancy
>congenital, acquired or a family history of disturbed bile secretion—*e.g.* the Dubin-Johnson and Rotor syndromes
>the occurrence of migraine and disturbed vision during the treatment

Special supervision is required in:

>a history of thrombophlebitis
>very pronounced varicosis
>epilepsy
>otosclerosis
>fibromyoma of the uterus
>hypertension with heart disease
>diabetes
>tetany
>porphyria

It must also be pointed out that existing acne can deteriorate slightly at the start of hormone treatment with any oestrogen and with cyclic progesterone-oestrogen administration and that results can only be expected from about the third month of treatment.

1. Oestrogens

Synthetic oestrogens: Stilbenes—non-steroidal synthetic oestrogens—now may no longer be used after animal experiments indicated an oncogenic potential, and are mentioned only for the sake of completeness. Strauss and Pochi [242] observed a favourable effect on acne under diethylstilboestrol at a dose of 0.5 mg/day for 3 weeks, starting with the 5th day of the cycle.

a) Oestriol (formula 4)

Oestriol is a degradation product of oestradiol and is eliminated with the urine. It stimulates the cervix and vaginal mucosa to proliferation even at low doses—1 to 2 mg/day—and is consequently

OESTRIOL   ETHINYL OESTRADIOL

Formulas 4 and 5

prescribed for female patients in the climacteric with pruritus of the vulva. Its effect on the endometrium, however, is extremely weak: proliferation is just recognizable at 20 mg/day [7, 187], so cycle disturbances and withdrawal bleeding are unlikely under this treatment.

A patient population of 54 females and 2 males received oestriol at a daily dose of 1–2 mg independent of the cycle. The results after 3 months of treatment were good in 62%, forms of acne with pronounced inflammation and those in which marked premenstrual exacerbation was present displaying the greatest improvement. In many cases it was also possible to maintain this success even after reducing the dosage to 2 mg daily from 10 days before menstruation. The side effects—one case each of postponement of menstruation and a sensation of tension in the breasts—were extremely low. An improvement of psychic mood was reported by many as an extremely positive side effect [51].

b) Conjugated Oestrogens

Conjugated oestrogens are sulphuric acid, or glucuronic acid-bound excretory forms of mainly animal oestrogens, *e.g.* oestrone sulphate, equiline sulphate, equilene sulphate, and likewise display only a slight effect on the endometrium. On administration of a dosage of 1–4 tablets of 125 mg/day from the 5th to the 23rd day of the cycle in a population of 137 patients, Lemke [131] observed very good results in 47.6% and good results in 38.7%. There were only occasional cases of intensified and prolonged menstrual bleeding and premenstrual spotting, but many cases of improved dysmenor-rhoeic complaints and premenstrual depression. Torre and Klump [249], who administered higher doses of conjugated oestrogens (1.25–8.75 mg) in the postovulatory phase only, achieved equally good results without inhibition of ovulation and without cycle disturbances.

c) Oestradiol

Oestradiol and its semisynthetic form, ethinyl oestradiol (formula 5) are the most potent oestrogens. The recommended mode of application is either oral administration of 0.02 mg ethinyl oestradiol cyclically in women and continuously in men [218] or i.m. injection of the depot preparation oestradiol valerate at a dosage of 10 mg at intervals of 4 weeks following menstruation [218] or at mid-cycle [210]. The results under the latter form of therapy are better than those observed under oestriol and conjugated oestrogens, being very good in 67% and good in 23%. However, when one considers that the physiological secretion rate of ovarian oestrogens during a cycle is 4–8 mg, then the dose administered appears to be relatively high. In keeping with this, the number of side effects was also much higher: in a population of 634 patients, cycle disturbances were recorded in 17%, while curettage was required in 0.5% because of excessive bleeding. Depot treatment with ethinyl oestradiol has also been performed in a male population. Gynaecomastia developed in 12 of the 369 cases, but this was found to be reversible and was regarded by the author to be negligible in comparison to the therapeutic results [210].

2. Oral Contraceptives

Many authors prefer the cyclical progestogenoestrogen therapy of acne in the form of oral contraceptives to the administration of oestrogens alone, since cycle disturbances and break-through bleeding are unlikely even at higher oestrogen doses [200, 267].

They also offer a further advantage in that they are suitable for female patients with acne vulgaris and a simultaneous desire for contraception [3, 11, 62, 136, 216, 238, 267, 278].

Apart from the so-called "mini-pill", which contains only a progestogen, oral contraceptives are combined preparations with oestrogenic and progestational hormones. A distinction is made between "monophasic preparations", the so-called "combined pills", which consist of 21 or 22 tablets containing a constant amount of progestogen and oestrogen, and "biphasic preparations". The latter—and particularly their modifications—were developed with the intention of imitating as closely as possible the hormonal situation of the normal cycle by means of exogenously administered steroids. Two versions are currently available on the market:

1. A preparation with which an oestrogen is administered alone in the first seven days, followed by 15 days with an oestrogen-progestogen combination,

2. Step-up pills, which contain just a slight amount of progestogen in addition to the oestrogen component on the first 11 days of the cycle. The dose of progestogen is increased somewhat in the second phase of the cycle (10 days) while the dose of oestrogen remains the same. Overall, however, they can be regarded as relatively oestrogen-dominant preparations because of the small amount of progestogen [125].

The oestrogens employed are either ethinyl oestradiol or mestranol, which have an identical, purely dose-dependent effect on the skin. In contrast, the progestogen component can exert greatly varying effects on the skin independent of the dose-effects which can become manifest even at low dosage in sensitive female patients. In particular, 19-nortestosterone and its derivatives display a pronounced androgenic partial effect.

That good results in the treatment of acne can nevertheless be achieved even with preparations of this composition is attributed on the one hand to the predominance of the oestrogenic effect and, on the other, to the central suppression of ovulation with physiologically increasing progesterone secretion [21] and ovarian androgen production. For example, a reduction of testosterone and androstenedione has also been observed under ovulation inhibitors containing 19-nortestosterone [76, 237].

Kümmel [127] achieved distinct improvement in patients with acne with an oral contraceptive containing 0.05 mg ethinyl oestradiol and 4 mg norethisterone. Strauss and Pochi [237] have reported exceptionally good results with a combination of ethinyl oestradiol or its 3-methyl ether mestranol and norethinodrel—likewise a 19-nortestosterone derivative. They also observed a significant decrease in the skin surface lipids following an initial slight increase of this parameter during the first two months of treatment. The oestrogen doses at 0.1–0.15 mg were, however, extremely high, particularly when one considers that the discovery of a risk of thromboembolic disease [81, 183] led to the recommendation that only oral contraceptives with a dose of ethinyl oestradiol of less than 50 mg should be prescribed.

This recommended reduction of the oestrogen dose is obviously a drawback in acne therapy—in sensitive patients in particular the androgenic partial effect of the progestogens can then abolish the oestrogen-induced inhibition of the sebaceous glands and even cause stimulation of sebaceous gland activity and induction or exacerbation of acne. This is also a possibility in the case of biphasic preparations, although a low total dose is generally administered here; the progestogen component is administered precisely in the second half of the cycle, *i.e.* in support of the physiological progestogen production, in order to achieve transformation of the endometrium similar to that in the normal cycle.

The use of antiandrogenic substances, such as megestrol acetate, chlormadinone acetate, and cyproterone acetate as the progestogen component, ensures a favourable therapeutic effect on acne even with low doses of oestrogen.

3. Antiandrogens: Cyproterone Acetate

Even preparations containing megestrol acetate or chlormadinone acetate as the progestogen component, which have a weaker antiandrogenic action, have been shown to be clearly superior to other oral contraceptives in their effect on the course of acne [137, 216, 268, 278].

The use of these two progestogen derivatives has been temporarily suspended due to the development of mammary tumours during long-term studies in beagle dogs.

However, tumours of this kind—which develop on the basis of hyperplasia of the entire mammary gland—can also be induced by progesterone in this animal species and—unlike in humans—17-α-hydroxyprogesterone esters in general have a much stronger progestational effect than derivatives of the 19-nortestosterone series. It must also be borne in mind that sex hormones can exert their effects at the level of the mammary gland only via interaction with pituitary hormones. Thus, the assumption that the tumorigenic effect of progestogens in the mammary gland is due to substance-specific influences is unfounded: no hyperplasia in any way comparable to that observed in the dog occurs in the human under therapeutic doses of progestogen [111, 157].

Much more pronounced is the antiandrogenic effect of 17-α-hydroxyprogesterone, or cyproterone acetate [156], which was synthesized by Wiechert in 1961 [263] and which is now regarded as the classical antiandrogen. In 1966, Neumann and Elger [156] observed a significant decrease in the size of the sebaceous glands in mature, castrated and testosterone-stimulated mice. In 1967, Archibal and Shuster demonstrated a significant decrease of sebum production in the rat after systemic therapy with cyproterone acetate.

Apart from its peripheral antiandrogenic effect, cyproterone acetate—unlike the free alcohol cyproterone—also has pronounced progestational and antigonadotropic effects (formulas 6 and 7) [86, 156]. The combination of these effects is of particular importance for the clinical use of antiandrogens, since, although the administration of a "pure" antiandrogen inhibits the effect of endogenous androgens, counter-regulatory mechanisms allow the "endogenous androgen deficit" thus induced to lead to intensified androgen production and secretion via gonadotropin stimulation. This situation is unlikely to occur on use of an antiandrogen of the cyproterone acetate type, since gonadotropin stimulation is antagonized as a result of the progestational effects [86].

CYPROTERONE

(1,2α-methylene-6-chloro-Δ^{4,6}
pregnadiene-17α-ol-3,20-dione)

CYPROTERONE ACETATE

(1,2α-methylene-6-chloro-Δ^{4,6}
pregnadiene-17α-ol-3,20-dione-
17α-acetate)

Formulas 6 and 7

To avoid the almost inevitable cycle disturbances, it was decided to administer cyproterone acetate combined with ethinyl oestradiol as an oral contraceptive, as a result of which the therapeutic inhibition of sebum production by the antiandrogen is further supported by the administration of oestrogens and inhibition of ovulation with its attendant lack of secretion of ovarian androgens and progesterone.

Hammerstein [92] recommended reverse sequential therapy: 100 mg cyproterone acetate/day for ten days, together with 0.04–0.06 mg ethinyl oestradiol/day for 21 days (Fig. 7). Using this dosage, many authors have observed a distinct regression of sebum secretion [270] and, hence, an improvement of the acne [137, 153, 268, 281]. Over and above this, marked signs of androgenization, *e.g.* hirsutism, were eliminated after about 6 to 9 months of treatment.

After a protracted period of use, however, the pronounced progestational effect at this high dosage leads to cycle disturbances in addition to occasional cases of loss of libido and signs of fatigue [132]; furthermore, amenorrhoea occurred after discontinuation of the therapy.

Since the potent antiandrogenic effect can occasionally also lead to pronounced drying-out of the skin as a result of the inhibition of sebum production, an attempt was made to make do with a lower dosage of cyproterone acetate—of approximately the same order as the progestogen component in conventional oral contraceptives [110, 128].

The results of these endeavours is the preparation SH B 209 AB [1], which contains 21 tablet of 2 mg cyproterone acetate combined with 50 μg ethinyl oestradiol in a calender pack. As with oral contraceptives, the tablets are taken from the 5th to the 25th day of the cycle;

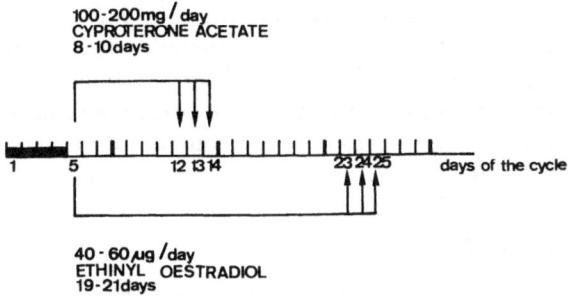

Fig. 7. Therapeutic regimen for cyproterone acetate by Hammerstein [92]

the next pack is started after a 7-day, tablet-free interval during which withdrawal bleeding occurs. 42 mg gestagen are therefore administered per cycle, whereby the transformation dosis of between 20 and 30 mg of this relatively strong progesterone derivative is only insignificantly exceeded [150].

Over 12,800 cycles in 1,350 females have shown the preparation to be a reliable contraceptive. Since no pregnancies occurred during this period of treatment, the 95% confidence limits for the Pearl index are 0.00–0.44. In a study lasting 12 months, mammography findings from females treated with SH B 209 AB were compared with those of an untreated control group. No clinically relevant differences were found between the findings of the two groups. Blood chemistry studies revealed slight changes, e.g. an increase of triglycerides, an increase of plasma insulin in the glucose tolerance test, an increase of plasma cortisol and an increase of plasma globulins, corresponding to those under other oral contraceptives [8].

The above-mentioned preparation was also investigated in an extensive clinico-therapeutic study in 80 acne patients, particular value being attached to a simultaneous dermatological and gynaecological assessment [48].

[1] Investigational preparation of Schering AG, Federal Republic of Germany: "Diane".

a) Clinico-Therapeutic Studies

Patients

   80 female patients with acne vulgaris and postpubertal acne were treated with
the combined preparation SH B 209 AB for 6 months and subjected to regular dermatological and gynaecological examinations. The age distribution of the patients
was between 16 and 39 years, with a mean age of 23.5 years. The acne had first
appeared between the ages of 11 and 33 years with an average of 16.3 years, and
the duration of the disease was 1½–21 years with an average of 7.3 years.

   The study population was chosen from patients presenting at an
acne clinic with primarily papulopustular lesions and premenstrual
exacerbation of the disease. The cases included several post-pubertal
forms of many years' standing, the history of which—*e.g.* premenstrual exacerbation, improvement during pregnancy, improvement or
exacerbation under the previous use of contraceptives, etc.—suggested
a hormonal influence.

Examinations and Therapy

   The severity of the clinical picture was assessed according to the
classification of Plewig and Kligman [176] before the start of treatment, the distribution being as follows:

First degree: 5 cases
Second degree: 22 cases
Third degree: 46 cases
Fourth degree: 7 cases

   All patients underwent a gynaecological examination and, in
additional to an assessment of the cycle pattern, determinations of
17-KS and OHCS in the 24-hour urine using the method of Apple-
bey-Norymberski [4] and determinations of serum testosterone by
means of radioimmunoassay were performed in 36 patients before the
start of treatment (normal values of 17-KS in mature women between 4.0 and 17.0 mg/24 hours, normal serum testosterone values
0.13–0.55 ng/ml serum).

   17-KS and OHCS values approaching the upper normal limit
for the average age of out female patients were found in only 3 subjects. Border-line serum testosterone values were found in 9 subjects
and distinctly increased values in 4 subjects.

   All patients received SH B 209 AB, the treatment scheme being
as described above. The only other concurrent therapy allowed in
the overwhelming majority of cases was inactive treatment (cleansing
of face with facial milk or facial water, use of indifferent ointment).

The results of the therapy were assessed as follows:

++ = very good = almost complete healing of the acne.
+   = good   = reduction of the inflammatory lesions by about 50%.
±   = moderate   = slight reduction of the inflammatory lesions, additional ther-
                   apy required.
0   = no effect.

Clinically, distinct degreasing of the skin and scalp hair and improvement of the acne were achieved in the majority of patients: the therapeutic results after a 6-month period of treatment were assessed as very good in 49 patients, good in 14 patients and moderate in 7 patients. 10 patients remained resistant to the therapy (Table 14).

Table 14. *Therapeutic results under treatment with SH B 209 AB [by Fanta (48)]*

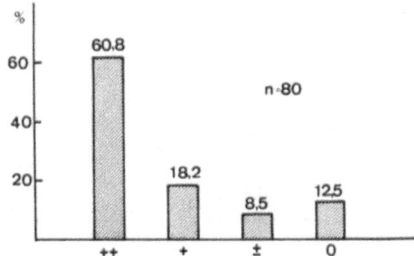

Thus, a distinctly positive effect which was fairly evenly distributed among the different degrees of acne was achieved in a total of 63 cases. Differences were, however, observed as regards the therapeutic response in relation to the clinical picture: the treatment was considerably less successful in the individual cases in which comedones predominated, while very good results were achieved in patients with pronounced papulopustular eruptions which had been relatively resistant to other therapeutic measures and which had also displayed marked premenstrual exacerbation (Ill. 24, 25).

An especially impressive finding was that all 12 patients with elevated or border-line serum testosterone values, all of whom were suffering from severe degrees of acne which had been resistant to therapy for many years, responded particularly well to the therapy, correlating with a reduction of serum testosterone values to normal values (Table 15). The different success ratings compared to other authors [150, 116], who report success and even complete healing in 96% of the cases as a result of the mentioned dosage of cyproterone acetate, is in the main probably due to differences in the patients chosen: most publications deal with primarily gynaecological patients *i.e.* with female patients who, in fact, were not seeking medical treatment primarily on account of acne but because they wished for a contraceptive. These patients, however, also happened to be suffering from acne.

The forms of acne resistant to therapy where immunological factors also play a part are rather to be found in dermatological patients.

The bleeding pattern was checked during administration of the combination SH B 209 AB and found to be very satisfactory. The interval between individual episodes of withdrawal bleeding was an

Table 15. *Therapeutic results under treatment with SH B 209 AB related to the serum testosterone values [by Fanta et al. (54)]*

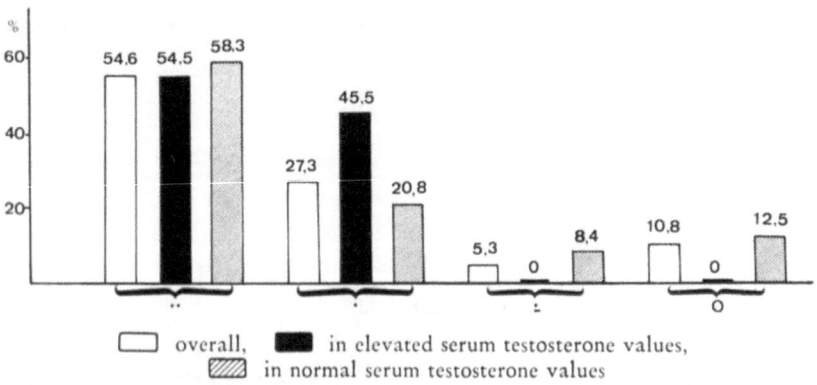

☐ overall,   ■ in elevated serum testosterone values,
▨ in normal serum testosterone values

average of 28 days with only slight deviations. No intermenstrual bleeding or break-through bleeding was observed. The rates for a largish population, referred to a total of 10,667 cycles without intake errors in female patients without a pertinent history, were as follows: spotting 1.5%, break-through bleeding 3.6%, spotting and break-through bleeding 0.7%. These figures are within the range of conventional combined preparations. The patients regarded the duration and intensity of bleeding as completely normal.

Side effects were reported by a total of 9 cases, nausea and breast tension being predominant and leading to discontinuation of the therapy in 4 patients at their request.

Dermatological follow-up examinations were performed in 40 cases for another 3–6 months after the end of therapy. 15 of these patients stopped using oral contraception altogether. The skin condition in 6 of these cases after an average of 4 months was still as good as at the end of therapy, whereas it had deteriorated again considerably in the other cases after just a short time.

At the end of a 6-month period of treatment with SH B 209 AB,

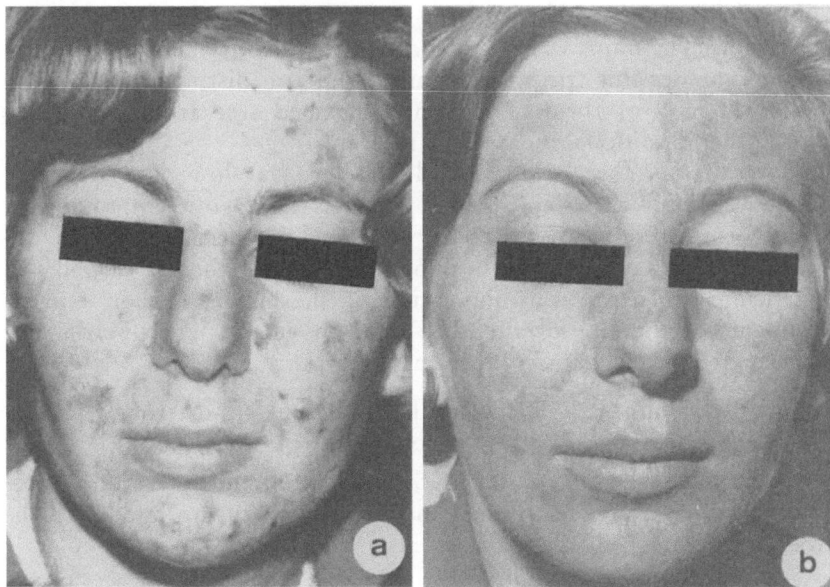

Ill. 24. Postpubertal progestational acne *a* before and *b* after six months' treatment with SH B 209 AB [54]

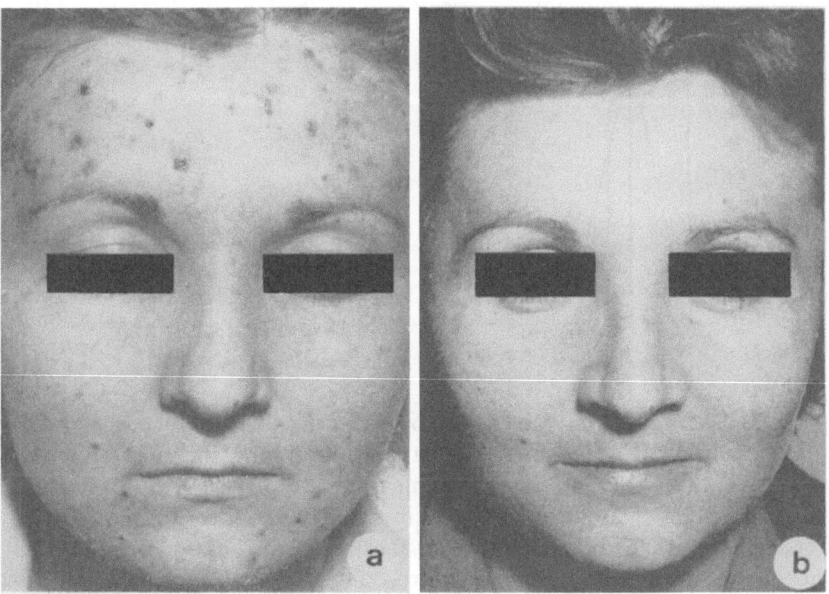

Ill. 25. Postpubertal progestational acne *a* before and *b* after 4 months' therapy with SH B 209 AB

25 patients were switched to a D-norgestrel-containing biphasic preparation. The improved skin condition was maintained in 8 of these patients under this treatment, while rapid and distinct deterioration occurred in 9 of them. 7 patients remained free from complaints with other, additional therapeutic measures.

It can therefore be concluded that, even at low dosage, cyproterone acetate can bring about a distinct therapeutic improvement. This form of therapy is especially indicated in patients with papulopustular forms of acne in late puberty or beyond the age of puberty, particular when there are indications in the history of hormone-dependent fluctuations of the acne and, above all, when border-line or elevated serum testosterone values are present.

b) Behaviour of 17-Ketosteroids and Serum Testosterone Under Cyproterone Acetate

Urinary 17-ketosteroid (17-KS) elimination and the serum testosterone values were determined in 25 patients during and after the therapy [54].

Table 16 a. *17-KS frequency distribution in patients with acne vulgaris before and after 6 months' treatment with SH B 209 AB: reduction of the mean values in the entire population (n = 25): x — 34%/o (* ▬▬ *), in patients with elevated ST values (n = 10): x — 31%/o (* ------ *) [by Fanta et al. (54)]*

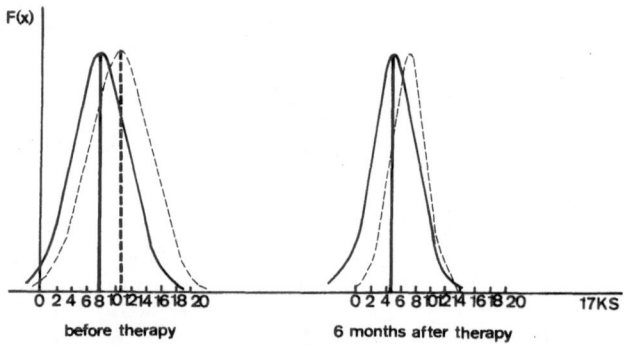

before therapy   6 months after therapy

17-KS elimination was found to be significantly reduced. Statistical evaluation of the frequency distribution among the entire population revealed a reduction of the mean value of 34%/o; a similar reduction (31%/o) was also observed in the 10 patients with primarily border-line to elevated serum testosterone values—they form part of the entire population. Furthermore, the graphic representation reveals compacting of the curves in accordance with the narrower scatter of the values (Table 16 a).

The reduction of the mean value in the serum testosterone frequency distribution was 28% for the entire population, and as high as 50% in patients with elevated initial values (Table 16 b). All findings were within the normal range after 6 months of treatment.

These results show that, in addition to the peripheral antiandrogenic effect, the chosen mode of administration—an ovulation inhibitor—also leads to suppression of ovarian androgen synthesis, so that an additional positive effect on the disease can be expected.

Table 16 b. *ST frequency distribution in patients with acne vulgaris before and after six months' treatment with SHB 209 AB: reduction of the mean values in the entire population:* $x_{25} — 27.5\%$ (▬▬▬), *in patients with elevated ST values;* $x_{10} — 50.3\%$ (------)

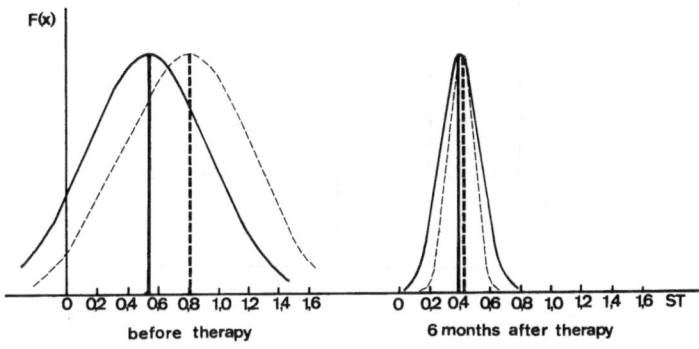

before therapy   6 months after therapy

c) Behaviour of the Skin Surface Lipids
Under Cyproterone Acetate

The casual level of skin surface lipids was determined before treatment with SH B 209 AB and after 3 months' treatment in 11 patients with an age distribution between 16 and 34 years and a mean age of 18 years [55]. The results show that the skin surface lipids were significantly reduced. The initial values varied between 0.5 and 2.3 mg/7 cm² with a mean of 1.5, while the final values varied between 0.3 and 1.7 with a mean of 0.8. The mean values were reduced by 45.7%. There was no change in the percental composition of the lipids on thin-layer chromatography. In most cases, the reduction of skin surface lipids was accompanied by a positive effect on the course of the disease.

In 3 subjects, the treatment was continued for a further month with a D-norgestrel-containing sequential preparation. Determination of the lipid values under this treatment revealed a distinct increase in all cases (Table 17).

The results of these studies—reduction of the serum testosterone values, reduction of skin surface lipids—corroborate the positive results obtained in the clinical study.

The good tolerance of this preparation and the reliable inhibition of ovulation justify the use of this form of therapy in particular in

Table 17. *Behaviour of skin surface lipids under 3 months' treatment with SH B 209 AB and a subsequent month's treatment with a biphasic preparation* □ ▲ ■ *[by Fanta and Müller (55)]*

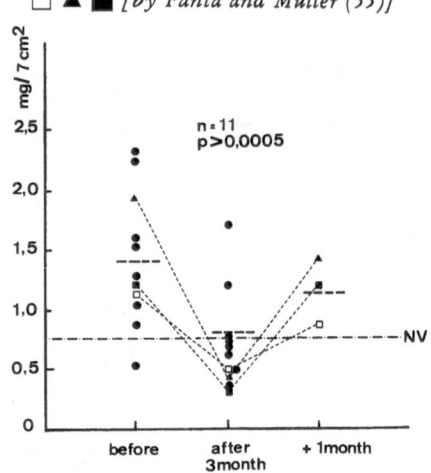

Statistical calculation using the t-test:

	before	after	
x̄	1.40	0.8	p > 0.005
σ	0.52	0.6	

cases with a desire for contraception and a concurrent disposition to acne. However, it also appears to be justified in all those cases in which premenstrual exacerbation cannot be prevented by other anti-acne agents.

4. Experimental Studies in Topical Hormone Therapy

Although systemic hormone therapy has meant a quite considerable advance in certain forms of acne, it represents significant intervention in the entire organism and must remain limited to a selected circle of patients. This fact led to the search for a topical hormone therapy in the hope of achieving many times the substance concentration present in the skin after oral administration and, at the same time, of avoiding systemic side effects as much as possible. The demands to be made of the ideal topical formulation are good penetration, direct inhibition of androgen stimulation of the sebaceous glands and low absorption or rapid inactivation of the active substance.

The first studies were directed towards the effect of topically applied oestrogens on the sebaceous glands. The results from animal experiments in castrated, androgen-stimulated rabbits were encouraging—topical use of a 17-β-oestradiol solution led to a significant reduction of the sebaceous gland volume [256]; however, the concentration chosen for the formulation—20%—was very high.

Further studies in human skin produced highly contradictory results which were not, however, attributable only to differences in the concentration and formulation—oestrogens are absorbed considerably better from a fatty ointment base—but also to discrepancies in the penetration and absorption of the individual metabolites. For example, oestriol penetrates considerably more slowly and to a lesser extent than the oestradiols and can be regarded as epidermotropic. On the other hand, the various oestradiols—17-α-oestradiol, which is virtually sex-unspecific, and the sex hormone 17-β-oestradiol—display almost identical penetration properties [259].

Individual reports of a decrease of sebum production after topical application of oestrogens vary greatly as regards the necessary concentration and the formulation [76, 265, 258]. However, they all agree that acne cannot be improved to any significant extent with concentrations which are unlikely to cause systemic side effects. This is understandable when one considers that the sebostatic effect of oestrogens is based primarily on a central effect and only partly on the still unclarified peripheral point of attack. The broad spectrum of action, which ranges from the epidermis via the hair follicle to the connective tissue, has led to the increasing use of oestrogen-containing topical agents in various other indications [168], e.g. male pattern alopecia [166], mammary aplasia, ulcus cruris, and diseases of the vaginal epithelium.

Topical application of progesterone in a 5% alcoholic solution resulted, in a double blind study, in a decrease in the sebum production, only, however, in the female patients tested; the male skin was unaffected [228]. It remains unclear, however, why the sebostatic effect, which was very marked in the initial months, completely was off after three months of treatment.

One could expect a considerably more potent effect on the sebaceous glands on topical application of cyproterone acetate; since, in contrast to oestrogens, the main factor with cyproterone acetate is the direct point of attack at the level of the skin, one can assume that a reduction of sebum production can be achieved with concentrations which have neither a progestational partial effect nor a general anti-androgenic effect.

In various series of studies, however, the substance has proved to be highly problematical with regard to stability, penetration, and absorption: a 10% cyproterone acetate-DMSO solution displayed just as weak an effect on the skin surface lipids of acne patients [35] as did a 5% solution in alcohol propylene glycol on the flank organ of Syrian hamsters [23]. The hypothetical assumption of a strong local sebostatic effect of cyproterone acetate has, however, been confirmed by means of another animal experiment: 3 weeks' treatment of the sebaceous glands in the internal ear of Syrian hamsters with a 2% cyproterone acetate-acetone solution, which was always made up immediately before use, brought about a statistically significant decrease of the labelling index and of the sebaceous gland volumes [135].

In this study, one ear was treated with the test solution, the other with pure acetone. A sebostatic effect was observed in both ears, although it was very much weaker in the ear treated with acetone. Whether this latter phenomenon was caused by a systemic effect of cyproterone acetate or by the acetone itself cannot be established because there was no untreated control ear.

In a personal series of studies we investigated the effect of an 0.5% cyproterone acetate solution in isopropanol/isopropylene myristat [2] (1 : 1, v/v) on animal models and patients [59].

First of all, the percutaneous absorption of intact human dorsal skin was studied using two direct methods—measuring the difference between the residues of labelled substance on the skin surface and in the stratum corneum after various exposure times, and determining the amount of activity eliminated via the urine up to 10 days after application [260]. A rapid decrease in the skin surface values and low urinary excretion permit the assumption of rapid penetration and a long tarrying time in the skin or extensive inactivation following absorption.

Comparative studies were also conducted with an 0.5% α-oestradiol solution in the same base and with the pure base.

a) Autoradiographic and Planimetric Studies in the Animal Model

The hamster ear model was chosen for this series of studies [177], since the sebaceous glands on the ventral side of the Syrian hamster ear are anatomically similar to the human sebaceous glands and are likewise androgen-sensitive.

A drop of the test solution (cyproterone acetate, 17-α-oestradiol or base) was applied to the inside of the right ear of each of 8 animals using a Pasteur pipette; the control ear of half of each group was treated with the base, but remained

[2] The formulation was donated by Schering AG, Berlin.

untreated in the other half. Four untreated animals served as the control group. The treatment lasted 3 weeks, after which autoradiography and histoplanimetry were performed *in vivo* using the methods described on page 6.

The results clearly illustrate the problems of developing a cyproterone acetate-containing topical agent:

Neither autoradiography nor histoplanimetry revealed any particular change in the sebaceous glands of the ears treated with cyproterone acetate or oestrogen. On the other hand, a distinct increase in the labelling indices was observed in the epidermis, follicular infundibulum, and sebaceous glands of the ears treated with the base; this was particularly significant in the follicular infundibulum— 14.5% compared to a control value of 10.8%. It is known that the sebaceous glands and follicular infundibula of the ventral side of the ears of various laboratory animals are particularly sensitive indicators of proliferation-activating stimuli. The present result therefore suggests that the vehicle—and isopropylene myristat is probably mainly responsible for this—masked any inhibitory effect of the active substance [72]. However, these studies have at least demonstrated that a systemic effect of the active substance can be ruled out, since no changes were observed in the untreated control ears of the animals treated on the test ear with cyproterone acetate or oestrogen.

b) Behaviour of Skin Surface Lipids

The behaviour of the skin surface lipids after 1 month's topical use of the 0.5% cyproterone acetate formulation was studied in 15 patients of both sexes with pronounced seborrhoea and papulopustular acne.

The patients were instructed to massage the solution well into the skin twice daily after cleansing with a milky lotion and water and not to use any other topical agents. Two further groups of 10 patients—one treated with the oestrogen formulation and the other with the base—were also studied.

The age distribution and severity of the disease were comparable in all three groups.

Lipid extraction and quantitative and qualitative determination of the lipids were performed according to the methods described on page 8.

A significant reduction of skin surface lipids almost to with the normal range, the extent of which with a fall of the mean values from 1.41 to 0.89 mg/cm^2 approached that of the fall in lipids after 3 months' treatment with SH B 209 AB, was observed after 1 month's topical treatment with cyproterone acetate (Table 18). The behaviour of the casual level of lipids and the replacement sum was virtually identical. The clinically very apparent degreasing of the skin surface

Therapy of Acne

Table 18. *Behaviour of skin surface lipids under 1 month's topical treatment with cyproterone acetate (0.5% in isopropanol/isopropylene myristat 1 : 1, v/v)*

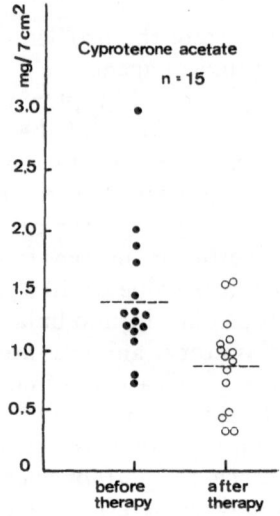

Statistical calculation using the t-test:

	before	after	
$\bar{x}$	1.41	0.83	$p > 0.0001$
σ	0.58	0.52	

Table 19. *Behaviour of skin surface lipids after 1 month's topical treatment with 17-α-oestradiol (0.5% in isopropanol/isopropylene myristat 1 : 1, v/v)*

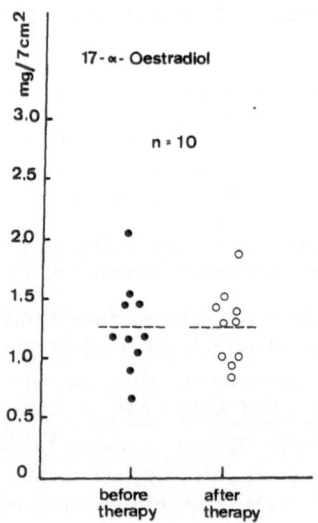

Table 20. *Behaviour of skin surface lipids after 1 month's use of isopropanol/ isopropylene myristat (1 : 1, v/v)*

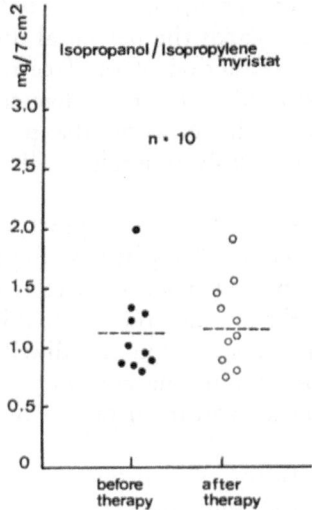

Table 21. *Decrease of free fatty acids under topical use of the base, cyproterone acetate and oestrogen solution (referred to 100°/o of the initial values)*

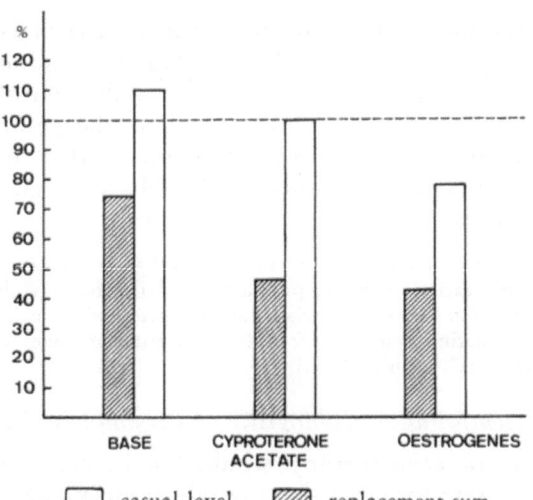

correlated well with this finding. At the same time, regression of the inflammatory lesions was also observed in most of the patients.

The values remained almost unchanged both in the oestrogen-treated group and in the group in which only the base was used (Tables 19 and 20). As regards the percental distribution of the individual lipid fractions, a reduction of the free fatty acid fraction was observed in all 3 groups of patients; a bacteriostatic effect of the isopropanol contained in the base on the propionibacterium acnes and, hence, inhibition of lipolysis might well be the reason for this (Table 21).

Although the sebostatic effect of topical treatment with cyproterone acetate might well be described as impressive and a further positive effect can be expected from the bacteriostatic property of the base, the findings from the animal studies should not be ignored.

Despite the fact that human skin is unlikely to be so sensitive to proliferation-activating stimuli, the currently used base could prove to be comedogenic after a protracted period of use and induce "cosmetic acne".

Thus, the topical efficacy of cyproterone acetate can be regarded as indisputable. The search must nevertheless continue for a formulation which is also suitable for clinical use and which takes account of every step in the multifactorial pathogenesis of acne.

D. Other Methods

1. Corticosteroids

Whereas the long-term systemic or topical use of corticosteroids can induce acneiform eruptions [109], short-term administration in severe nodulocystic acne rapidly leads to a reduction of the inflammatory component [200]. It should, perhaps, be pointed out again here that Pochi and Strauss [181] have observed that the administration of glucocorticoids also supports the sebaceous gland-inhibitory effect of oestrogens.

The treatment for acute inflammatory exacerbation of severe nodulocystic acne is oral administration of 40 mg prednisolone daily for 7–10 days, or a single intramuscular injection of 40 mg triamcinolone acetonide, or the intralesional application to fluctuating cysts of a few drops of triamcinolone acetonide diluted with physiological NaCl solution [200].

2. Other Attempts at Antiphlogistic and Immunological Therapy

The picture of acne therapy would not be complete without a description of a few forms of therapy which individual authors have recently attempted in primarily severe, inflammatory acne. The mechanism of action of some of these modalities is unknown; the therapeutic results are mainly restricted to a small population or are highly contradictory.

a) Sulfones

The administration of sulfones can lead to satisfactory improvement in about 50% of cases of severe, inflammatory forms of acne and conglobate acne [113]. Like sulfonamides—to which they are related—sulfones also have a bacteriostatic property. However, their efficacy in acne is attributable not so much to this as to an antiphlogistic effect brought about via stabilization of the lysozymes.

Plewig and Kligman [176] recommend their use in combination with antibiotics and desquamative agents at a dosage of 100 mg/day in the first week followed by an increase to 200 mg/day which is then maintained until the inflammation regresses markedly—this may take several months. The haemogram must be monitored during the therapy, since—apart from methaemoglobin formation, which does not require discontinuation of the therapy—haemolysis and, although extremely rarely, leucopenia and agranulocytosis can occur. Other side effects are gastrointestinal complaints and allergic and toxic exanthem.

b) Zinc

The observation that a deficit of zinc following longterm parenteral feeding leads to sebaceous gland hyperplasia with the occurrence of seborrhoeic lesions and acneiform eruptions [114] has prompted some researchers to try zinc therapy in inflammatory forms of acne.

The hypothetical assumptions regarding the mechanism of action are, on the one hand, that zinc is a major factor in the activation of 20 enzyme systems—including the 17-β-hydroxysteroid dehydrogenase, which is involved in testosterone and oestrogen metabolism—and a deficit of zinc could therefore result in decelerated break-down of androgenic substances [28] and, on the other, that zinc stabilizes macromolecules and biological membranes and affects the migration rate and phagocytosis activity of macrophages [30]. Zinc is, however, on the other hand a strong stimulator in the production of a substance corresponding to the prostaglandin E, and it is possible that a certain prostaglandin deficiency could play a part in the acne [102]. Accordingly, it could intervene in the dynamics of the inflammatory process and reduce the inflammatory component of acne.

For acne therapy, Michaelsson [145] recommends a dosage of 0.2 g zinc sulphate 3 times daily, which is the equivalent of 125 mg zinc. However, whereas Michaelsson [145] observed significant results with this zinc therapy in comparison to placebo in a double-blind study in 54 patients, the finding is contradicted by the results of Weisman [257], who found that zinc therapy had no positive effect at all on the disease. Cunliffe and Ma. [37], for example, achieved positive results in cases of severe pustular acne.

c) Hyposensitization and Active Immunization

Since the structure of acne lesions suggests the involvement of infection-allergic processes, Stickl *et al.* [232] attempted to influence the disease immunologically via hyposensitization and active immunization. Basing on their knowledge of the "oral enteral tolerance reaction" gained in animal experiments, they chose an oral form of administration using lyophilized propionibacteirum acnes as the antigen. A success rate of 80% was achieved with this therapy in a population of 117 patients with inflammatory forms of acne.

d) Levamisole

Levamisole is a polycyclic broad-spectrum anthelmintic which has been shown in *vivo* and *in vitro* studies to stimulate reduced cell-mediated hypersensitivity reactions of the delayed type [77, 246] and which has since been employed above all in chronic bacterial, mycotic, and viral infections, and in cancer. Isolated reports indicate good results in conglobate acne as well [105].

3. UV

One can almost conclude from clinical observations that ultra-violet light has a positive effect on acne: many patients report a considerable improvement of the complaint in the summer months, followed, however, by a deterioration in the cooler months. In particular, inflammatory lesions on the upper part of the body disappear after exposure to sunlight. For this reason, ray treatment using instruments with a selected ultra-violet spectrum has been increasingly used in recent years in acne therapy. Properly conducted studies, however, do not yet exist and the therapeutic mechanism too remains unclear. In view of the proven comedogenic effect of actinic irritation and the still unknown causal factor of acne aestivalis, this method of treatment should still be very carefully examined. It is possible that ultra-violet rays have, in the first instance, an anti-inflammatory and also anti-microbial effect but also act as a stimulus to the formation of new comedones so that the acne flares up again more seriously at a later date.

4. Cosmetics

The existence of detergent acne on the one hand [147] and cosmetic acne on the other [122] means that patients must be warned against both over-dramatic cleansing measures and the excessive use of cosmetic preparations, even if the latter enjoy the name of "acne cosmetics". Excessive washing with strong degreasing detergents and mask-like camouflaging of the lesions are expressions of the mental distress of acne patients, but must at the same time be regarded as a disturbing factor in the healing process of acne.

Milky emulsions or low-alcohol tonics are recommended for skin cleansing, and make-up should only be used by way of exception. An "acne toilet" with mechanical removal of open comedones following facial steam baths appears to be advisable not only from a psychological point of view [200]—it can, for example, also considerably reduce pustular eruption in the initial stages of vitamin A acid therapy. However, a certain dexterity is required for good results; treatment by a well-trained beautician with gentle use of a ventouse is definitely to be preferred to the frequently heavy-handed self-treatment by the patient.

5. Diet

There is still no documented proof of the effect of the diet on the pathogenesis of acne [97, 70], although foodstuffs have frequently been quoted as provoking factors [33, 38, 67]. Chocolate has been blamed above all else, but attempts to exacerbate existing acne through excessive consumption of chocolate have failed [70, 66].

The recent interpretation of acne as a food allergy [162] has also been refuted [276]. Allergy tests for various food allergens performed in 120 patients produced a negative result in 80%. The observance of an elimination diet in the patients with positive reactions had no effect at all on the acne.

6. Psychological Management

Although recent years have seen the development of extremely effective acne therapy, the psychological management of the patients should not be neglected. Most of the patients are in their puberty and the disease, which is seen by other age groups as a trivial matter, is regarded by them as a severe handicap. Since it is difficult for them to find the necessary patience for effective acne therapy, it is essential for them to be informed at the start of treatment that no acne therapy can be expected to lead to satisfactory results within less than 2–3 months, that recurrences are possible even under properly conducted therapy and that, once the desired result is achieved, it can only be upheld by long-term maintenance therapy.

IV. Conclusion

The development of modern anti-acne agents is based on the knowledge so far gained of the many causes and the pathogenesis of this disease, and on differentiation of the many forms of acne.

The topical use of retinoic acid and benzoyl peroxide and systemic long-term treatment with antibiotics are now well acknowledged and firmly established modes of treatment. A significant extension of the therapeutic spectrum can be expected from intervention in the hormonal regulation of the sebaceous glands and in the immune system.

A favourable effect can be achieved in many cases of acne by the administration of oestrogens. Far superior to this, however, is the systemic administration of the antiandrogen cyproterone acetate in the form of an oral contraceptive: the use of this modality—which still represents major intervention in the complex regulatory mechanism of the body—is justified in specific indications, e.g. premenstrual and postpubertal forms of acne, a desire for contraception with a simultaneous disposition to acne, and can be regarded as a quite considerable advance in these cases.

Since, however, treatment with hormones and especially with anti androgens in their present form of administration must remain restricted to a selected group of patients, the search for further sebosuppressive agents continuous to be urgent. There have recently been reports on a strong anti-androgenic and thereby anti-seborrhoeic effect of the H_2-receptor-antagonistic cimetidin. Its use in acne therapy is, however, still contraversial in as far as its anti-androgenic effect is not restricted in the sebaceous glands but, at least in animal experiments, affects all androgen-dependent organs.

Very good results have been achieved, particularly in the case of conglobate acne, by therapy with 13-Cis retinoic acid: 13 out of 14 patients were cured after 4 months of treatment and the positive outcome continued even after termination of the therapy. As points of attack, on the one hand, a selective, i.e., non-hormonal sebo-suppression, on the other, prevention of keratinization. Side effects in the form of a xerosis, cheilitis and drying up of the nasal mucous are, however, frequent and additional tests on the toxicity must be carried out. Further, experiments on guinea-pigs and hamsters using the topical application of 17-alpha-porpyltestosterone [62] resulted in a reduction in the size of the sebaceous gland probably through nullifying the effect of dihydrotestosterone; the untreated side remaining uneffected. Even in the case of systematic dosage, other androgene-dependent organs were only affected when the dosage reached the high level of 100 mg/kg.

The decision as to whether a non-hormonal sebo-suppressive or a topical-effective hormonal antiandrogen without systematic effect [114, 138], for example by incorporating cyproterone into a base which is suitable for clinical use, represents the optimal therapeutic agent for acne in the future, will only be able to be made after numerous further experimental and clinical tests.

References

1. Adlam, C., Scott, M. T.: Lymphoreticular stimulatory properties of coryne-bacterium parcum and related bacteria. Med. Microbiol. *6*, 261 (1973).
2. Agache, P., Barrand, Ch., Colette, Cl., Raffi, A., Laurent, R.: Sebum levels during the first year of life. European Symposium of Dermato-logical Research Amsterdam (April 1976).
3. Amann, W., Spanknebel, G.: Rückbildung von Akne vulgaris bei Gabe eines Antikonzipiens. Zschr. Haut- u. Geschlkrkh. *36*, 225 (1974).
4. Appelbey, J. I., Gibson, G., Norymberski, J. K., Stubbs, R. D.: Indirect analysis of corticosteroids. Bioch. J. *60*, 453—460 (1955).
5. Archibal, A., Shuster, S.: Bioassay of androgen using the rat sebaceous gland. J. Endocr. *37*, 22 (1967).
6. Aron-Brunetière, R.: An attempt at a physiopathological explanation of seborrhea and acne vulgaris: Therapeutic results. Brit. J. Dermat. *65*, 157—164 (1953).
7. Artner, J., Gitsch, E.: Über Lokalwirkungen von Östriol. Geburtshilfe und Frauenheilkunde *19*, 812—819 (1959).
8. Aydinlik, S., Lachnit-Fixson, U.: Diane — eine Gestagen-Oestrogen-Kombi-nation mit Antiandrogenwirkung. Med. Monatsschr. *31*, 425—429 (1977).
9. Baer, R. L., Leshaw, S. M., Shalita, A. R.: High-dose tetrazykline therapy in severe acne. Arch. Derm. *112*, 479 (1976).
10. Bailey, N., Pinneau, S. R.: Tables for predicting adult height from skeletal age: Revised for use with Greulich-Pyle hand standards. J. Pediat. *40*, 423—441 (1952).
11. Barfield, W. E.: Acne successfully treated by inhibition of ovulation. J. Amer. Med. Ass. *201*, 30 (1967).
12. Basler, R. S. W.: Potential hazards of clindamycin in acne therapy. Arch. Derm. *112*, 383 (1976).
13. Beck, A.: The oestrogenic and progestagenic of oral contraceptives—clinical and pharmakological aspects. 3. Seminario internazionale sul controllo della fecondita, Genova, 3.—5. Marzo 1977.
14. Berch, H. v. d.: Studien über Porphyrin. Dtsch. Med. Wschr. *36*, 1492—1494 (1928).
15. Berlin, G.: Acne comedo in children due to paraffinoil applied on the head. Arch. Derm. Suppl. *69*, 683—687 (1954).
16. Blank, I. H.: Factors which influence the water content of the stratum cor-neum. J. Invest. Dermatol. *18*, 433—440 (1952).
17. Blank, I. H., Gould, E.: Penetration of anionic surfactants into skin. J. Invest. Dermatol. *37*, 311—315 (1961).
18. Bonne, C., Raynaud, J.-P.: Characterization and hormonal control of the androgen receptor in the hamster sebaceous glands. J. Invest. Dermatol. *68*, 215—220 (1977).
19. Bonne, C., Saurat, J.-H., Chivot, M., Lehuchet, D., Raynaud, J.-P., Androgen receptor in human skin. Br. J. Dermatol. *97*, 501—503 (1977).
20. Braun-Falco, O., Lincke, H.: Zur Frage der Vitamin B_6-/B_{12}-Akne. Ein Bei-trag zur Acne medicamentosa. Münch. med. Wschr. *118*, 155—160 (1976).

21. Briggs, M. Briggs, M.: Plasma hormone concentrations in women receiving steroid contraceptives. J. Obstet. Gynaecol. Br. Commonw. *79*, 946—950 (1972).
22. Bues, M.: Die Roteigenfluoreszenz des Gesichtes und der Mundhöhle. Dissertation, Kiel 1976.
23. Burdick, K. H., Hill, R.: The topical effect of the antiandrogen chlormadinone acetate and some of its chemical modifications on the hamster costo-vertebral organ. Br. J. Dermatol. Suppl. *6*, 19—25 (1970).
24. Burtenshaw, J. M. L.: The mortality of hemolytic streptococcus on the skin and other surfaces. J. Hyg. *38*, 575 (1938).
25. Burton, J. L., Shuster, S.: The relationship between seborrhea and acne vulgaris. Br. J. Dermatol. *84*, 600—601 (1971).
26. Burton, J. L., Laschet, V., Shuster, S.: Reduction of sebum excretion in man by the antiandrogen cyproterone acetate. Br. J. Dermatol. *89*, 487—490 (1973).
27. Calman, K. C.: Androgens and acne: A new method for the screening of antiandrogens in human skin. Br. J. Dermatol. *82*, Suppl. 6, 26—33 (1970).
28. Calman, K. C., Muir, A. V., Hilne, J. A.: Survey of distribution of steroid dehydrogenases in sebaceous glands of human skin. Br. J. Dermatol. *82*, 567—571 (1966).
29. Caplan, R. M.: Gynecomastia from a nonestrogenic anti-androgen. J. Clin. Endocrin. *27*, 1348—1349 (1967).
30. Chvapil, M.: New aspects in the biological role of zinc: A stabilizer of macromolecules and biological membranes. Life Sci. *13*, 1041 (1975).
31. Cohen, L. K., George, W., Smith, R.: Isoniazid-induced acne and pellagra. Occurrence in slow inactivators of isoniazid. Arch. Derm. *109*, 377—381 (1974).
32. Col, W., Akers, A., Maibach, H. I.: Relative safety of long-term administration of tetracycline in acne vulgaris. Cutis *17*, 531—539 (1976).
33. Cormia, F. E.: Food sensitivity as a factor in the etiology of acne vulgaris. J. Allergy *12*, 34 (1940).
34. Cummins, C. S., Johnson, J. L.: Corynebacterium parvum: A synonym for propionibacterium acnes? J. Gen. Microbiol. *80*, 433—442 (1974).
35. Cunliffe, W. J., Shuster, S., Smith, A. J.: The effect of topical cyproterone acetate on sebum secretion in patients with acne. Br. J. Dermatol. *81*, 200—201 (1969).
36. Cunliffe, W. J., Cotterill, J. A.: The acnes—Major problems in dermatology. London-Philadelphia-Toronto: W. B. Saunders. 1975.
37. Cunliffe, W. J., Burke, B., Dodman, B., Gould, D. J.: A double-blind trial of a zinc sulphate/citrate complex and tetracycline in the treatment of acne vulgaris. Br. J. Dermatol. *101*, 321 (1979).
38. Cunningham, T. D., Mendenhall, J. C.: Observations on acne and allergy. J. Allergy *7*, 378 (1936).
39. Downing, D. T., Strauss, J. S., Pochi, P. E.: Variability in the chemical composition of human skin surface lipids. J. Invest. Derm. *53*, 322—327 (1969).
40. Ebling, F. J.: Factors influencing the response of the sebaceous glands of the rat to androgen. Br. J. Dermatol. *82*, Suppl. 6, 10—15 (1970).
41. Ebling, F. J.: Hormonal control of the sebaceous gland in experimental animals. In: Advances in biology of skin, Vol. 4: Sebaceous glands (Montagna, W., Ellis, R. A., Silver, A. F., eds.), pp. 200. Oxford: Pergamon Press. 1973.

42. Ebling, F. J.: Hormonal control and methods of measuring sebaceous gland. J. Invest. Dermatol. 62, 161—171 (1974).
43. Ebling, F. J.: The role of the pituitary in acne. Cutis 17, 469—474 (1976).
44. Ebling, F. J., Ebling, E., McCaffery, V., Skinner, J.: The responses of the sebaceous glands of the hypophysectomized-castrated male rat to 5-α-androstanedion and 5-α-androstane-3-β, 17-diol. J. Invest. Dermatol. 60, 183—187 (1973).
45. Elias, P. M., Goerke, J., Friend, D. S.: Mammalian epidermal barrier layer lipids: composition and influence on structure. J. Invest. Dermatol. 69, 535—547 (1977).
46. Erb, W., Böhle, E.: Investigation of fecal lipids by thin-layer. Z. klin. Chem. klin. Biochem. 6, 379—383 (1968).
47. Esposito, C.: Acne neonatorum. Gi. e. Miss. Derm. 110, 393—394 (1975).
48. Fanta, D.: Oral contraceptives in dermatology. International Symposium on Hormonal Contraception, Excerpta Medica, Utrecht, September 1977.
49. Fanta, D.: Tetrazyklintherapie der Akne. Der Prakt. Arzt 370, 281—286 (1978).
50. Fanta, D.: Klinische und experimentelle Untersuchungen über die Wirkung von Benzoylperoxid in der Behandlung der Akne. Hautarzt 29, 481—486 (1978).
51. Fanta, D., Stöger, H.: Hormontherapie der Akne vulgaris. Wien. klin. Wschr. 87, 158—163 (1975).
52. Fanta, D., Niebauer, G.: Aktinische (senile) Komedonen. Z. H. + G. 51, 791—797 (1976).
53. Fanta, D., Bardach, H., Jurecka, W.: Klinische Erfahrungen mit Benzoylperoxid in der Behandlung der Acne vulgaris. Wien. klin. Wschr. 89, 748—750 (1977).
54. Fanta, D., Schneider, W. H. F., Spona, J., Neufeld, T.: Die Anwendung von Antiandrogenen in der Behandlung der Akne. Wien. klin. Wschr. 89, 622—627 (1977).
55. Fanta, D., Müller, M. M.: Effect of Cyproteronacetate on skin surface lipids. Acta derm. venerol. 58, 86—87 (1978).
56. Fanta, D., Müller, M. M.: Effect of benzoylperoxide on skin surface lipids. Dermatologica 158, 55—59 (1978).
57. Fanta, D., Formanek, I., Poitschek, Ch., Thurner, J.: Porphyrinproduktion des Propionibacterium acnes bei Akne und Seborrhoe. Arch. Derm. 261, 175—179 (1978).
58. Fanta, D., Jurecka, W.: Autoradiographic investigations in benzoylperoxide treated skin. Acta Dermatoven. 2, 361—363 (1978).
59. Fanta, D., Jurecka, W., Müller, M. M., Ramadan, W.: Effects of topical application of cyproteronacetat and estrogens on skin surface lipids (in Vorbereitung).
60. Fanta, D., Spona, J.: Serumtestosteronwerte bei Patientinnen mit Akne vulgaris (unpublizierte Ergebnisse).
61. Farnsworth, W. E., Brown, J. R.: Metabolism of testosterone by the human prostate. J.A.M.A. 183, 436—439 (1963).
62. Ferrari, R. A., Chakrabarty, K., Beyler, A. L., Wiland, J.: Suppression of sebaceous gland development in laboratory animals by 17α-propyltestosteron. J. Invest. Derm. 71, 320—323 (1978).
63. Fisher, A. A.: The safety of topical erythromycin. Contact Dermat. 2, 43—44 (1976).

64. Forest, M. G., Cathiard, A. M., Bertrand, J. A.: Evidence of testicular activity in early infancy. Rapid Communications *37*, 148—151 (1973).
65. Formanek, J., Fanta, D., Poitschek, Ch., Thurner, J.: Porphyrinproduktion des Propionibacterium Acnes. Arch. Derm. Res. *259*, 169—176 (1977).
66. Förström, L., Mustakallio, K. K., Dessypris, A., Uggeldahl, P. E., Adler-creutz, H.: Plasma testosterone levels and acne. Acta Dermatoven. *54*, 369—371 (1974).
67. Frank, S. B.: Acne vulgaris. Springfield, Ill.: Charles C Thomas. 1971.
68. Frey, L., Ramsey, C. A.: Tetracycline in acne vulgaris: clinical evaluation and the effect on sebum production. Br. J. Dermatol. *78*, 653—700 (1966).
69. Frost, P., Gomez, E. C.: Inhibitors of sex hormones: development of experimental models. In: Advances in biology of skin; pharmacology and the skin (Montagna, W., Van Scott, E., Stoughton, R. B., eds.), pp. 403—420. New York: Appleton, Century-Crofts. 1972.
70. Fulton, J. E., Plewig, G., Kligman, A. M.: Effect of chocolate on acne vulgaris. J. Amer. med. Ass. *210*, 2071 (1969).
71. Fulton, J. E., jr., Pablo, G.: Topical antibacterial therapy for acne. Arch. Derm. *110*, 83—86 (1974).
72. Fulton, J. E., Farzad-Bakshandeh, A., Bradley, S.: Studies on the mechanism of action of topical benzoylperoxide and vitamin A acid in acne vulgaris. J. Cutan. Pat. *1*, 191—200 (1974).
73. Fulton, J. E., Bradley, S., Aqundez, A., Black, Th.: Non-comedogenic cosmetics. Cutis *17*, 344—351 (1976).
74. Gallegos, A. J., Berliner, D. L.: Transformation and cojugation of dehydroepiandrosterone by human skin. J. Clin. Endocrinol. *27*, 1214—1218 (1967).
75. Gitsch, E., Schneider, W. H. F., Spona, J.: Radioisotope in Geburtshilfe und Gynäkologie. Berlin-New York: Walter de Gruyter. 1977.
76. Givens, J. R., Andersen, R. N., Wiser, W. L., Umstot, E. S., Fish, S. A.: The effectiveness of two oral contraceptives in suppressing plasma androstenedione, testosterone, LH, and FSH, and in stimulating plasma testosterone-binding capacity in hirsute women. Amer. J. Obstet. Gynecol. *124*, 333—339 (1976).
77. Glogan, R., Spitler, L., Nelms, D., O'Connor, R., Olson, J., Ostler, P., Silverman, S., Smolin, G.: Clinical and immunologic effects of levamisole. Clin. Res. *23*, 291 A (1973).
78. Gloor, R., Hübscher, M., Friederich, H. C.: Untersuchungen zur externen Behandlung der Akne vulgaris mit Tetracyclin und Oestrogenen. Hautarzt *25*, 391—394 (1974).
79. Gloor, M., Hummel, A., Friederich, H. C.: Experimentelle Untersuchungen zur Benzoylperoxidtherapie der Acne vulgaris. Z. H. + G. *50*, 657—663 (1975).
80. Gloor, M., Klump, K., Wirth, H.: Cytocinetic studies of the sebosuppressive effect of drugs using the example of benzoyl-peroxide (in Vorbereitung).
81. Goldzieher, J. W., Dozier, T. S.: Oral contraceptives and thromboembolism: a reassessment. Amer. J. Obstet. Gynec. *123*, 878—914 (1975).
82. Gomez, E. C., Hsia, S. L.: *In vitro* metabolism of testosterone-4-^{14}-C and 4'-androstene-3,17-dione-4-^{14} C in human skin. Biochemistry *7*, 24—32 (1968).
83. Götz, H., Reichenberger, M., Zabel, G.: Untersuchungen über die Akne vulgaris bei 2249 Oberschülern im Alter von 12 bis 20 Jahren. Schrift. Marchionini Stftg. *2*, 25—42 (1971).
84. Gould, D., Cunliffe, W. J., Holland, K. T.: Chemotaxis and acne. European Symposium of Dermatological Research, Amsterdam 1976.

85. Gowland, G., Ingham, E., Holland, K. T., Cunliffe, W. J.: P. acnes hyaluronidase: purification and properties. European Symposium of Dermatological Research, Amsterdam 1976.

86. Gräf, K.-J., Neumann, F.: Klinische Anwendungsmöglichkeiten von Antiandrogenen in der Dermatologie. Ärztl. Kosmetologie 6, 26—27 (1976).

87. Grant, J. D., Anderson, P. C.: Chocolate as a cause of acne: A dissenting view. Missouri Med. 62, 459 (1965).

88. Greene, R. S., Downing, D. T., Pochi, P. E., Strauss, J. S.: Anatomical variation in the amount and composition of human skin surface lipid. J. Invest. Dermatol. 51, 240—247 (1970).

89. Hägele, W., Schäfer, H., Stüttgen, G.: Über die Bedeutung der Triglyceridspaltung durch Corynebacterium acnes für die Acne vulgaris. Arch. Derm. Forsch. 246, 328—334 (1973).

90. Hamilton, J. B.: Male hormone substance. A prime factor in acne. J. Clin. Endocrin. 1, 570—592 (1941).

91. Hamilton, J. B., Montagna, W.: The sebaceous glands of the hamster: I. morphological effects of androgenes on integumentary structures. Am. J. Anat. 86, 191—234 (1950).

92. Hammerstein, J., Cupceancu, B.: Behandlung des Hirsutismus mit Cyproteronacetat. Dtsch. Med. Wschr. 94, 829—834 (1969).

93. Haskin, D., Lasher, N., Rothman, S.: Some effects of ACTH, cortisone, progesterone and testosterone on sebaceous glands in the white rat. J. Invest. Dermatol. 20, 207—212 (1953).

94. Hay, J. B., Hodgins, M. B.: Metabolism of androgens by human skin in acne. Br. J. Dermatol. 91, 123—133 (1974).

95. Herrmann, F., Prose, P. H., Sulzberger, M. B.: Studies on the ethersoluble substances on the human skin. J. Invest. Dermatol. 21, 397—419 (1953).

96. Hitch, J. M.: Acneform eruptions induced by drugs and chemicals. J. Amer. med. Ass. 200, 879—880 (1967).

97. Hitch, J. M., Greenburg, E. G.: Adolescent acne and dietary iodine. Arch. Derm. 84, 898—911 (1969).

98. Hodgson-Jones, I. S., MacKenna, R. M. B., Wheatley, V. R.: The study of human sebaceous activity. Acta Dermatoven. 32, Suppl. 29, 155—161 (1952).

99. Hofmann, C., Plewig, G., Braun-Falco, O.: Ungewöhnliche Nebenwirkungen bei oraler Photochemotherapie (PUVA-Therapie) der Psoriasis. Hautarzt 28, 583—588 (1977).

100. Hong Lioe Ko, Heczko, P. B., Pulverer, G.: Differential susceptibility of propionibacterium acnes, P. granulosum and p. avidum to free fatty acids. J. Invest. Dermatol. 71, 363—366 (1978).

101. Hooker, C. W., Pfeiffer, C. A.: Effects of sex hormones upon body growth, skin, hair and sebaceous glands in the rat. Endocrinology 32, 69—76 (1943).

102. Horrobin, D. F., Karmazyn, M., Manku, M. S., Karmali, R. A., Morgan, R. O., Ally, A. I.: Zinc, acrodermatitis, acne and prostaglandin. Br. Med. J. 191 (1977).

103. Hsia, S. L., Voigt, W.: Inhibition of dihydrotestosterone formation an effective means of blocking androgen action in hamster sebaceous gland. J. Invest. Dermatol. 62, 224—227 (1974).

104. Imamura, S., Pochi, P. E., Strauss, J. S., McCabes, W. R.: The localization and distribution of corynebacterium acnes and its antigens in normal skin and the lesions of acne vulgaris. J. Invest. Dermatol. 53, 143—150 (1969).

105. Ippen, H., Quadripur, S. A.: Levamisol zur Behandlung von Hautkrankheiten. Dtsch. Med. Wschr. 100, 1710—1711 (1975).

106. Izumi, A. K., Marples, R. R., Kligman, A. M.: The bacteriology of acne comedones. Arch. Derm. *102*, 397—399 (1970).
107. Johnson, O. R.: Treatment of acne in the female with a hormone. J. Maine M. A. *42*, 258 (1951).
108. Jurecka, W., Fanta, D.: Autoradiographische Untersuchungen an aktinischen (senilen) Komedonen. Arch. Derm. Res. *260*, 81—86 (1977).
109. Kaidbey, K. H., Kligman, A. M.: The pathogenesis of topical steroid acne. J. Invest. Dermatol. *62*, 31—36 (1974).
110. Kaiser, E., Loch, E. G., Winckelmann, G., Schröpfl, F., Dietz, M., Hartmann, P.: Behandlung mit Antiandrogenen bei der Frau. Med. Welt *27*, 1836—1841 (1976).
111. Kaiser, R.: Gestagenanwendung bei Genital- und Mammatumoren. Stuttgart: G. Thieme. 1973.
112. Kalz, F., Scott, A.: Cutaneous changes during the menstrual cycle. A. M. A. Arch. Derm. *74*, 493—503 (1956).
113. Kaminsky, C. A., Kaminsky, A. R. de, Schicci, C., Morini, M. V. de: Acne: Treatment with diaminophenylsulfone. Cutis *13*, 869—871 (1974).
114. Katchen, B., Dancik, St., Millington, G.: Percutaneous penetration and metabolism of topical ^{14}C-flutamide in men. J. Dermatol. *66*, 379—382 (1976).
115. Kay, R. G., Tosman-Jones, C., Pybus, J., Whiting, R.: A syndrome of acute zinc deficiency during total parenteral alimentation in man. Am. Surg. *183*, 331 (1976).
116. Keller, P. J., Fetz, A., Schär, A., Floersheim, Y.: Behandlung von Akne und Seborrhoe mit Antiandrogenen. Schweiz. med. Wschr. *108*, 1640—1642 (1978).
117. Kelly, P., Burns, R. E.: Akute febrile ulcerative conglobate acne with polyarthralgy. Arch. Derm. *104*, 182—187 (1971).
118. Kirschbaum, J. O., Kligman, A. M.: The pathogenetic role of corynebacterium acnes in acne vulgaris. Arch. Derm. *88*, 832—833 (1963).
119. Kligman, A. M.: An overview of acne. J. Invest. Dermatol. *62*, 268—287 (1974).
120. Kligman, A. M.: The uses of the sebum? In: Advances in biology of skin: The sebaceous glands, Vol. IV, 110—124 (1962).
121. Kligman, A. M., Fulton, J. E., Plewig, G.: Topical vitamin A acid in acne vulgaris. Arch. Derm. *99*, 469—476 (1969).
122. Kligman, A. M., Mills, O. H.: Acne cosmetica. Arch. Derm. *106*, 843—850 (1972).
123. Kligman, A. M., Plewig, G.: Classification of acne. Cutis *17*, 520—522 (1976).
124. Knutson, A.: Ultrastructural observations in acne vulgaris. The normal sebaceous follicle and acne lesion. J. Invest. Dermatol. *62*, 288—307 (1974).
125. Kopera, H.: Kontrazeption mit einem normophasischen Präparat. Wien. med. Wschr. *127*, 573—577 (1977).
126. Krause, W.: Gonadotropine, Testosteron und Östradiol im Plasma bei Acne vulgaris. Der Hautarzt *28*, 368—370 (1977).
127. Kümmel, J.: Beeinflussung der Akne vulgaris durch Ovulationshemmer. Med. Welt *17*, 138—139 (1966).
128. Lachnit-Fixson, U., Kaufmann, J.: Zur Beeinflußung von Androgenisierungserscheinungen. Med. Klin. *72*, 1922—1926 (1977).
129. Lasher, N., Lorincz, A. L., Rothman, S.: Hormonal effectson sebaceous glands in the white rat. III. Evidence for the presence of a pituitary sebaceous gland tropic factor. J. Invest. Dermatol. *24*, 499—505 (1955).
130. Lee, P. A.: Acne and serum androgens during puberty. Arch. Derm. (Chic.) *112*, 482—485 (1976).

131. Lemke, G.: Beitrag zur Hormonbehandlung der Akne vulgaris bei weiblichen Kranken. Z. H. + G. 47, 501—508 (1972).

132. Leo-Rossberg, I., Laur, S., Zielske, F., Hammerstein, J.: Reversed sequential therapy of hirsutism using cyproteroneacetate. Acta endocr. Suppl. 152, 14 (1971).

133. Leyden, J. J., McGinley, K. J., Mills, O. H., Kligman, A. M.: Propionibacterium levels in patients with and without acne vulgaris. Invest. Dermatol. 65, 382—384 (1975).

134. Lim, L. S., James, V. H. T.: Plasma androgens in acne vulgaris. Br. J. Dermatol. 91, 135—143 (1974).

135. Luderschmidt, Ch., Plewig, G.: Effects of cyproterone acetate and carboxylic acid derivates on the sebaceous glands of the Syrian hamster. Arch. Derm. Res. 258, 185—191 (1977).

136. Ludwig, E.: Ovulationshemmer und Akne. In: Ovulationshemmer in der Dermatologie (Zaun, H. O., ed.). Stuttgart: G. Thieme. 1972.

137. Ludwig, E.: Über die Anwendung cyproteronacetathältiger Ovulationshemmer in der Dermatologie. Kongreßbericht, 30. Tag. d. Dtsch. Dermatolog. Ges. Graz, 1974.

138. Lutsky, B. N., Budak, M., Koziol, P., Monahan, M., Neri, R. O.: The effects of a nonsteroid antiandrogen, flutamide, on sebaceous gland activity. J. Invest. Dermatol. 64, 412—417 (1975).

139. Marples, R. R., Downing, D. T., Kligman, A. M.: Control of free fatty acids in human skin surface lipids by corynebacterium acnes. J. Invest. Dermatol. 56, 127—131 (1971).

140. Matoltsy, A. G., Matoltsy, M. N.: Cytoplasmic droplets of pathologic horny cells. J. Invest. Dermatol. 38, 323—325 (1962).

141. Mauvais-Jarvis, P., Charransol, G., Bobas-Masson, F.: Simultaneous determination of urinary androstanediol and testosterone of human androgenicity. J. Clin. Endocrinol. Metab. 36, 452—459 (1973).

142. Mayr-Rohn, J.: Mikrobiologie der Akne. Ärztl. Kosmetologie 6, 132—134 (1976).

143. Meigel, W. N., Prückner, H.: Therapie der Akne vulgaris mit PanOxyl. Z. Hautkr. 52, 725—732 (1977).

144. Meinhof, W., Kaiser, E., Loch, E.-G.: Die androgenetische Akne der Frau. Der Hautarzt 25, 34—38 (1974).

145. Michaelsson, G., Juhlin, L., Vahlquist, A.: Effect of oral zink and vitamin A in acne. Arch. Dermat. 113, 31 (1977).

146. Miescher, G., Schönberg, A.: Untersuchungen über die Funktion der Talgdrüsen. Bull. schweiz. Akad. med. Wissensch. 1, 101—114 (1944).

147. Mills, O. H., Kligman, A. M.: Acne detergicans. Arch. Derm. 111, 65—68 (1975).

148. Mills, O. H., Kligman, A. M., Stewart, R.: The clinical effectiveness of topical erythromycin in acne vulgaris. Cutis 15, 93 (1975).

149. Morales, A., Pujari, B.: The choice of estrogen preparations in the treatment of prostatic cancer. Canad. Med. Ass. 113, 865—867 (1975).

150. Moltz, L., Meckies, J., Hammerstein, J.: Die kontrazeptive Betreuung androgenisierter Frauen mit einem niedrig dosierten cyproteronacetathältigen Einphasenpräparat. Dtsch. med. Wschr. 104, 1376—1382 (1979).

151. Morello, A. M., Downing, D. T., Strauss, I. S.: Octadecadienoic acids in the skin surface lipids of acne patients and normal subjects. J. Invest. Dermatol. 66, 319—323 (1966).

152. Münzberger, H., Reichel, K., Niebauer, G., Gschwandtner, W. R.: Einfluß von Umweltstrahlung auf die Prophyrinrotfluoreszenz des Gesichtes. Ann. Ital. di Derm. Clin. e Sper. *28*, 195—202 (1974).

153. Neale, Ch., Krebs, D., Bettendorf, G.: Behandlung der Akne, des Hirsutismus und der Alopezie mit Cyproteron-Acetat und Äthinyl-Oestradiol. Acta endocr. Suppl. *152*, 13 (1971).

154. Nelson, R. M., Rakoff, A. E.: Hirsutism and acne treated by an androgen antagonist. Obstetrics and Gynecol. *5*, 748—752 (1970).

155. Neumann, F.: Chemische Konstitution und pharmakologische Wirkung. In: Die Gestagene — Handb. d. exp. Pharmakologie, Vol. 22/1, ch. VI (Junkmann, K., ed.), pp. 680—1025. Berlin-Heidelberg-New York: Springer. 1974.

156. Neumann, F., Elger, W.: The effect of a new antiandrogenic steroid 6-chloro-17 hydroxy-1α, 2α-methylenepregna-4,6-diene-3,20-dione acetate (cyproterone acetate) on the sebaceous glands of mice. J. Invest. Dermatol. *46*, 461—572 (1966).

157. Neumann, F., Elger, W., Salloch, R. H: Wirkung von Gestagen auf äußeres Genitale, Cervix, Uterus, Tube, Ovar und Hoden. In: Die Gestagene I — Handb. d. exp. Pharmakologie (Junkmann, K., ed.), p. 50. Berlin-Heidelberg-New York: Springer. 1969.

158. Newman, B. A., Feldman, F. F.: Adult premenstrual acne. A. M. A. arch. Derm. + Syph. *69*, 356—363 (1954).

159. Niebauer, G., Ebner, H.: Zur elektronenmikroskopischen Darstellung der Keratinosomen (Odland-Körper) mit Hilfe der Osmium-Zinkjodid-Methode. Cytobiologie *1*, 322—327 (1970).

160. Niebauer, G., Gschwandtner, W. R., Reichel, K., Münzenberger, H.: Über die Eigenfluoreszenz der Haut. Vortrag anläßlich d. 1. Jahressitzung der ARD, Düsseldorf, 24./25. 11. 1973.

161. Niermann, H.: Bericht über 230 Zwillinge mit Hautkrankheiten. Z. menschl. Vererb. Konstit. Lehre *34*, 483 (1958).

162. Obeid, V.: Akne und Ernährung. Vortrag anläßlich der 57. Jahresversammlung der Schweiz. Gesell. Dermat. u. Venerol. 17./18. 10. 1975. Refer. in: Medical Tribune *9*, Nr. 4 (1976).

163. Oertel, G. W., Schirazi, M., Hoffmann, G.: Bestimmung von cAMP im Plasma während des Zyklus und in der Menopause. Abstract. 216, 40. Tagung Dtsch. Ges. Gyn. Gebh., Wiesbaden 24./28. 9. 1974.

164. O'Malley, B. P., Anderson, I., Rosenthal, R. D.: Bone lesions in systemic acne. Br. J. Dermatol. *100*, 703 (1979).

165. Orentreich, N., Durr, N.: The natural evolution of comedones into inflammatory papules and pustules. J. Invest. Dermatol. *62*, 316 (1974).

166. Orfanos, C. E., Wüstner, H.: Penetration und Nebenwirkungen lokaler Östrogenapplikation bei Alopecia androgenetica. Hautarzt *26*, 367—369 (1975).

167. Pace, W. E., A benzoylperoxide-sulfur cream for acne vulgaris. Canad. Med. An. J. *93*, 252—254 (1965).

168. Panteleos, D., Orfanos, C. E.: Die Aufnahme und therapeutische Anwendung von lokal appliziertem Östrogen. Ärztl. Kosmetologie *6*, 159—163 (1976).

169. Peck, G. L., Olsen, G. Th., Yoder, F. W., Strauss, J. S., Downing, D. T., Panpya, M., Butkus, D., Arnaud-Battandier, J.: Prolonged remissions of cystic and conglobate acne with 13-cis-retinoic acid. New Engl. J. Med. *300*, 329—333 (1979).

170. Plewig, G.: Acne vulgaris: Proliferative cells in sebaceous glands. Br. J. Dermatol. *90*, 623—630 (1974).

171. Plewig, G.: Klassifikation und Ätiopathogenese der Akne. In: Fortschritte der praktischen Dermatologie und Venerologie, Vol. 8 (Braun-Falco, O., Marghescu, S., eds.). Berlin-Heidelberg-New York: Springer. 1976.

172. Plewig, G.: Alterungsvorgänge der Talgdrüsen. Ärztl. Kosmetologie 6, 1—8 (1976).

173. Plewig, G., Christophers, E., Braun-Falco, O.: Proliferative cells in the human sebaveous gland. Acta Dermatovener. (Stockholm) 51, 413—422 (1971).

174. Plewig, G., Kligman, A. M.: Induction of acne by topical steroids. Arch. Derm. Forsch. 247, 29—52 (1973).

175. Plewig, G., Schöpf, E.: Antiinflammatory effects of antimicrobial agents: an in vivo study. J. Invest. Dermatol. 65, 532—536 (1975).

176. Plewig, G., Kligman, A. M.: Acne—morphogenesis and treatment. Berlin-Heidelberg-New York: Springer. 1975.

177. Plewig, G., Luderschmidt, Ch.: Hamster ear model for sebaceous glands. J. Invest. Dermatol. 68, 171—176 (1977).

178. Pochi, P. E.: Acne in premature ovarian failure, reestablishment of cyclic flare-ups with medroxyprogesterone acetate therapy. Arch. Derm. 109, 556—557 (1974).

179. Pochi, P. E., Strauss, J. S., Rao, G. S., Sarda, I. R., Forchielli, E., Dorfman, R. I.: Plasma testosterone and estrogen levels, urine testosterone excretion and sebum production in males with acne vulgaris. J. Clin. Endocr. 25, 1660—1664 (1965).

180. Pochi, P. E., Strauss, J. S.: Endocrinologic control of the development and activity of the human sebaceous glands. J. Invest. Dermatol. 62, 191—201 (1974).

181. Pochi, P. E., Strauss, J. S.: Sebaceous gland inhibition from combined glucocorticoid-estrogen treatment. Arch. Derm. 112, 1108—1109 (1976).

182. Pochi, P. E., Strauss, J. S., Downing, D. T.: Skin surface lipid composition, acne, pubertal development and urinary excretion of testosterone and 17-ketosteroids in children. J. Invest. Dermatol. 69, 485—489 (1977).

183. Preston, S. N.: The oral contraceptive controversy. Amer. J. Obstet. Gynec. 111, 994—1007 (1971).

184. Pria, S. D., Greenblatt, R. B., Mahesh, V. B.: An antiandrogen in acne and idiopathic hirsutism. J. Invest. Dermatol. 52, 348—350 (1969).

185. Price, V. H.: Testosterone metabolism in the skin. Arch. Derm. 111, 1496—1502 (1975).

186. Puccinelli, V. A., Califano, A.: Contributo alla conoscenza della struttura e della formazione del comedone. G. Ital. Dermatol. 106, 235—248 (1965).

187. Puck, A.: Die Wirkung von Oestrol bei Dysmenorrhoe, Entzündungen im weiblichen Genitale, Pruritus und Beschwerden der Klimax. Münch. Med. Wschr. 99, 1505—1507 (1957).

188. Puhvel, S. M.: Dermal hypersensitivity of patients with acne vulgaris to corynebacterium acnes. J. Invest. Dermatol. 49, 154—158 (1967).

189. Puhvel, S. M., Acne from an immunological perspective. Cutis 17, 502—507 (1976).

190. Puhvel, S. M., Barfatani, M., Warnick, M., Sternberg, T. H.: Study of antibody levels to corynebacterium acnes. Arch. Derm. 90, 421—427 (1964).

191. Puhvel, S. M., Warnick, M. A., Sternberg, T. H.: Levels of antibody to staphylococcus epidermidis in patients with acne vulgaris. Arch. Derm. 92, 88—90 (1965).

192. Puhvel, S. M., Sakamoto, M.: A Reevaluation of Fatty Acids as inflammatory agents in acne. J. Invest. Dermatol. *68*, 93—97 (1977).
193. Puhvel, S. M., Amirian, D., Weintraub, J., Reisner, R. M.: Lymphocyte transformation in subjects with nodulo-cystic acne. Br. J. Dermatol. *97*, 205—211 (1977).
194. Puhvel, S. M., Sakamoto, M.: An *in vivo* evaluation of the inflammatory effect of purified comedonal components in human skin. J. Invest. Dermatol. *69*, 401—406 (1977).
195. Punnonen, R.: Effect of castration and peroral estrogen therapy on skin. Acta Obstet. Gynec. Scand. *51*, Suppl. 21, 32 (1972).
196. Rajka, G.: Delayed reactivity to bacterial and viral extracts in different dermatosis. Acta Dermatoven. *50*, 281—286 (1970).
197. Ray, L. F., Kellum, R. E.: Corynebacterium acnes from Human Skin. Arch. Derm. *101*, 36—40 (1970).
198. Rassner, G., Scherwitz, E.: Akne — Sonderformen. In: Fortschritte der praktischen Dermatologie und Venerologie, Vol. 8, pp. 297—303. Berlin-Heidelberg-New York: Springer. 1976.
199. Reid, M. R., Altemeyr, W. A.: Peroxide ointments. Ann. of Surgery *118*, 741—749 (1943).
200. Reisner, R. M.: The rational therapy of acne. Cutis *17*, 527—530 (1976).
201. Reiss, F., Gellis, S.: Effects produced on the pilosebaceous and the adrenals of the rabbit by inunction of sex hormones. J. Invest. Dermatol. *12*, 159—172 (1949).
202. Resh, W., Stoughton, R. B.: Topically applied antibiotics in acne vulgaris. Arch. Derm. *112*, 182 (1976).
203. Revesz, C., Chappel, C. I., Gaudry, R.: Masculinization of female fetuses in the rat by progestational compounds. Endocrinology *66*, 140—144 (1960).
204. Ricketts, C. R., Squire, J. R., Topley, E., Lilly, H. A.: Human skin lipids with particular reference to the self-sterilizing power of the skin. Clin. Sci. *10*, 89 (1951).
205. Rimington, C., Magnus, I. A., Ryan, E. A., Cripps, D. S.: Porphyria and photosensitivity. Q. J. Med. *36*, 29—57 (1967).
206. Rongone, E. L.: Testosterone metabolism by human male mammary skin. Steroids *7*, 489—504 (1966).
207. Rony, H. R., Zakon, S. J.: Effect of androgen on the sebaceous glands of human skin. Arch. Derm. Syph. *48*, 601—604 (1943).
208. Rothman, S.: Physiology and biochemistry of the skin. Chicago: Univ. of Chicago Press. 1954.
209. Rothman, S., Smiljanic, A., Shapiro, A. L., Wettkamp, A. W.: The spontaneous cure of tinea capitis in puberty. J. Invest. Derm. *8*, 81—98 (1947).
210. Ruhrmann, H.: Hat die Hormontherapie der Acne in ihren verschiedenen Erscheinungsformen noch einen Sinn? Der Hautarzt *26*, 140—143 (1975).
211. Ruhrmann, H., Schulten, K. H.: Über das quantitative Verhalten der Hautoberflächenlipide vor und nach i. m. Injektion hoher Dosen von Depot-Testosteron. Arch. klin. exp. Derm. *211*, 224—229 (1960).
212. Sansone, G., Reisner, R. M.: Differential rates of conversion of testosterone to dihydrotestosterone in acne and in normal human skin: A possible pathogenic factor in acne. J. Invest. Dermatol. *56*, 366—372 (1971).
213. Schaefer, H.: The quantitative differentiation of sebum excretion using physical methods. J. Soc. Cosmetic Chem. *24*, 331—353 (1973).
214. Scheibenreiter, S.: Acne infantum. Z. f. Kinderheilkunde *99*, 195—198 (1967).

215. Schirren, C. G., Honsig, C. H.: Über die Lipidregenerationszeit im Bereich talgdrüsenfreier Haut. Hautarzt *19*, 53—56 (1969).
216. Schirren, C. G., Immel, L.: Hormonale Therapie der Akne vulgaris: Ovulationshemmer bei prämenstrueller Akne. Münch. Med. Wschr. *111*, 1742—1747 (1969).
217. Schreus, H. Th.: Zur Pathogenese und Therapie der Akne conglobata. Z. Haut-u. Geschl. Krk. *16*, 1—4 (1954).
218. Schreus, H. Th.: Fortschritte in der hormonellen Therapie der Akne. Der Hautarzt *18*, 70—73 (1967).
219. Scott, D. G., Cunliffe, W. J., Gowland, G.: Activation of complement— a mechanism for the inflammation of Acne. Br. J. Dermatol. *101*, 315 (1979).
220. Schumacher, A., Stüttgen, G.: Vitamin-A-Säure bei Hyperkeratosen, epithelialen Tumoren und Akne. Orale und lokale Anwendung. Dtsch. med. Wschr. *40* 547 (1971).
221. Scott, M. T.: Biological effects of the adjuvant corynebacterium parvum: II. Evidence for macrophage T-cell interaction. Cell. Immunol. *5*, 465 (1972).
222. Shahrad, W., Marks, R.: A Pharmacological effect of oestrone on human epidermis. Br. J. Dermatol. *97*, 383—386 (1977).
223. Shalita, A. R., Wheatley, V. R.: Inhibition of pancreatic lipase by tetracycline. J. Invest. Dermatol. *54*, 413—415 (1970).
224. Shehadeh, N. H., Kligman, A. M.: The bacteriology of acne. Arch. Derm. *88*, 829—831 (1973).
225. Shuster, S.: The bioassay of androgen, anti-androgen and other hormones on the sebaceous gland. Br. J. Dermatol., Suppl. 6, 15—19 (1970).
226. Shuster, S., Thoday, A. J.: The control and measurement of sebum secretion. J. Invest. Dermatol. *62*, 172—190 (1974).
227. Siemens, H. W.: Die Vererbungspathologie der Akne. Münch. Med. Wschr. *73*, 1514—1517 (1926).
228. Simpson, N. B., Bowden, B. E., Forster, A., Cunliffe, W. J.: The Effect of topically applied progesterone on sebum excretionsrate. Br. J. Dermatol. *100*, 687 (1969).
229. Smith, M. A., Waterworth, P. M.: The bacteriology of acne vulgaris in relation to the treatment with antibiotics. Br. J. Dermatol. *73*, 152—159 (1961).
230. Sönnichsen, N., Jakobza, D., Hackenberg, C.: Akne conglobata mit Arthralgie und Allgemeinsymptomen. Dermatol. Monatsschr. *163*, 835—839 (1977).
231. Spona, J.: Rapid assay for luteinizing hormone and evaluation of data by a new computer program. In: Radioimmunoassay and related procedures in medicine, Vol. 1, pp. 123—130. Vienna: Intern. Atomic Energy Agency. 1974.
232. Stickl, H., Hüllstrung, H. W., Gillesberger, W.: Akne vulgaris. Immunbiologische Behandlung. Archiv. d. prakt. Med. *7*, 161—162 (1975).
233. Strauss, J. S., Kligman, A. M.: The effect of ACTH and hydrocortisone on the human sebaceous gland. J. Invest. Dermatol. *33*, 9—14 (1959).
234. Strauss, J. S., Kligman, A. M.: The pathologic dynamics of acne vulgaris. Arch. Derm. *82*, 779—790 (1960).
235. Strauss, J. S., Kligman, A. M., Pochi, P. E.: The effect of androgens and estrogens on human sebaceous glands. J. Invest. Dermatol. *39*, 139—155 (1962).
236. Strauss, J. S., Pochi, P. E.: Effect of enovid on sebum production in females. Arch. Derm. *87*, 366—368 (1963).
237. Strauss, J. S., Pochi, P. E.: Effect of cyclic progestin—estrogen therapy on sebum and acne in women. J.A.M.A. *190*, 815—819 (1964).

238. Strauss, J. S., Pochi, P. E.: Intracutaneous injection of sebum and comedones. Arch. Derm. *92*, 443—454 (1965).

239. Strauss, J. S., Pochi, P. E., Sarda, I. R., Wotiz, H. H.: Effect of oral and topical 17-alpha-methyl-B-nortestosterone on sebum production and plasma testosterone. J. Invest. Dermatol. *52*, 95—99 (1969).

240. Strauss, J. S., Pochi, P. E.: Assay of anti-androgens in man by the sebaceous gland response. Br. J. Dermatol. *82*, Suppl. 6, 33—43 (1970).

241. Strauss, J. S., Pochi, P. E.: Effect of cyclic-estrogen therapy on sebum and acne in women. J.A.M.A. *190*, 470—477 (1971).

242. Strauss, J. S., Pochi, P. E., Downing, D. T.: The role of skin lipids in acne. Cutis *17*, 485—487 (1976).

243. Stüttgen, G.: Zur Lokalbehandlung von Keratosen mit Vitamin-A-Säure. Dermatologica (Basel) *124*, 65—80 (1962).

244. Stüttgen, G., Schaefer, H.: Funktionelle Dermatologie. Berlin-Heidelberg-New York: Springer. 1974.

245. Sullivan, M., Zeligman, I.: Acneform eruption due to corticotropin. A.M.A. Arch. Derm. *73*, 133—141 (1956).

246. Symoens, J.: Levamisole: An anti-anergic chemotherapeutic agent, an overview December 1975. Second international Conference on Modulation of Health. The J. E. Fogarty Internat. Center and Nat. Cancer Inst., Bethesda, Maryland, December 1975.

247. Thody, A. J., Shuster, S.: The effects of hypophysectomy and testosterone on the activity of the sebaceous glands of castrated rats. J. Endocrinol. *47*, 219—224 (1970).

248. Thyresson, N.: Acne conglobata and septicemia. Acta Dermatoven. *43*, 496—499 (1963).

249. Torre, D., Klumpp, M. M.: Cyclic estrogenic hormone therapy of acne vulgaris. J.A.M.A. *164*, 1447—1449 (1957).

250. Ufer, J.: Hormontherapie in der Frauenheilkunde. Berlin-New York: Walter De Gruyter. 1972.

251. Unna, P. J.: Die Histopathologie der Hautkrankheiten. Berlin: A. Hirschwald 1894.

252. Vasarinsh, P.: Benzoylperoxid-sulfur lotion. Arch. Derm. *98*, 133—186 (1968).

253. Voigt, W., Fernandez, E. P., Hsia, S. L.: Transformation of testosterone into 17 β-hydroxy-5α-androstan-3 one by microsomal preparations of human skin. J. Biol. Chem. *245*, 5594—5599 (1970).

254. Voigt, W., Hsia, S. L.: Further studies on testosterone 5-α-reductase of human skin: Structural features of steroid inhibitors. J. Biol. Chem. *248*, 4280—4285 (1973).

255. Weinstock, M., Wilgram, G. F.: Fine structural observations on the formation and enzymatic activity of keratinosomes in mouse tongue filiform papilae. J. Ultrastruct. Res. *30*, 262—274 (1970).

256. Weirich, G., Longauer, J.: Inhibition of sebaceous glands by topical application of oestrogen and anti-androgen on the auricular skin of rabbits. Arch. Derm. Forsch. *250*, 81—93 (1974).

257. Weisman, K., Wadskov, S., Søndergaard, J.: Oral zinc sulfate therapy for acne vulgaris. Acta Dermatoven. *57*, 357—360 (1977).

258. Weitgasser, H.: Beitrag zur modernen Aknetherapie. Z. H. + G. *38*, 261—267 (1965).

259. Wendker, H., Schaefer, H., Zesch, A.: Penetrationskinetik zur Verteilung lokal applizierter Östrogene. Arch. Derm. Forsch. *256*, 67 (1976).

260. Wendt, H.: Resorptionsstudie mit Cyproteronacetat. Persönliche Mitteilung.

261. Wheatley, V. R.: Sebum, Lipogenesis and Acne. Cutis *17*, 475—485 (1976).

262. Whiteside, J. A., Voss, J. G.: Incidence and lipolytic activity of propionibacterium acnes and p. granulomatosum. (II) in acne and in normal skin. J. Invest. Dermatol. *60*, 94—97 (1973).

263. Wiechert, R., Neumann, F.: Gestagene Wirksamkeit von 1-Methyl- und 1,2-Methylen-Steroiden. Arzneimittelforsch. *15*, 244—246 (1965).

264. Wilson, J. D.: Recent studies on the mechanism of action of testosterone. New Engl. J. Med. *287*, 1284—1291 (1972).

265. Wilson, J. D., Walker, J. D.: The conversion of testosterone to 5-androstan-17-β-ol-3-one (dihydrotestosterone) by skin slices of man. J. Clin. Invest. *48*, 371—379 (1969).

266. Winkler, K.: Die Antiandrogene in der Dermatologie (Gravimetrische Fettbestimmung während Cyproteronanwendung). Arch. klin. exp. Derm. *233*, 296—302 (1968).

267. Winkler, K.: Orale Kontrazeptiva und Akne vulgaris. Hautarzt *23*, 241—243 (1972).

268. Winkler, K.: Antiandrogene bei Akne vulgaris. Hautarzt *26*, 661—662 (1975).

269. Winkler, K.: Innerliche Behandlung der Akne mit Hormonen. In: Fortschritte der praktischen Dermatologie und Venerologie, Vol. 8 (Braun-Falco, O., Marghescu, S., eds.). Berlin-Heidelberg-New York: Springer. 1976.

270. Winkler, K., Schaefer, H.: Das Verhalten der Talgsekretion während der Behandlung der Acne mit Cyproteronacetat und Athinylöstradiol. Arch. Dermatol. Forsch. *247*, 259—264 (1973).

271. Wolff, K., Holubar, K.: Odland-Körper (Membrane Coating Granules. Keratinosomen) als epidermale Lysosomen. — Ein elektronenmikroskopischcytochemischer Beitrag zum Verhornungsprozeß der Haut. Arch. Klin. Exp. Dermatol. *231*, 1—19 (1967).

272. Wolff, H. H., Braun-Falco, O., Christophers, E.: Die Wirkung von Vitamin-A-Säure auf die Epidermis. Autoradiographische, histologische und elektronenmikroskopische Untersuchungen. Acta histochem. (Suppl.) 183 (1970).

273. Wolff-Schreiner, E., Stingl, G.: Vitamin-A-Säure-Behandlung der Acne vulgaris. Überblick über Ergebnisse und praktische Erfahrungen. Hautarzt *26*, 460—465 (1975).

274. Woodbury, L. P., Lorincz, A. L., Ortega, P.: Studies on pituitary sebotropic activity. II. Further purification of a pituitary preparation with sebotropic activity. J. Invest. Dermatol. *45*, 364—367 (1965 b).

275. Wotiz, H. H., Mescon, H., Doppel, H., Lemon, H. M.: The *in vitro* metabolism of testosterone by human skin. J. Invest. Dermatol. *26*, 113—119 (1956).

276. Wüthrich, B., Much, Th.: Akne vulgaris: Ergebnis einer Nahrungsmittel-Allergen-Testung und einer kontrollierten Eliminations-Diät. Acta Dermatol. *3*, 177—183 (1977).

277. Zarate, A., Mahesh, V. B., Greenblatt, R. B.: Effect of an Antiandrogen, 17-methyl-B-nortestosterone, on acne and hirsutism. J. Clin. Endocr. Metab. *26*, 1394—1398 (1966).

278. Zaun, H.: Systemische Therapie mit Sexualhormonen in der dermatologischen Praxis. Acta Dermatol. *2*, 33—38 (1976).

279. Zelick, R.: Antibiotics. In: Diseases of medical progress: A study of iatrogenic disease (Moser, R. H., ed.). Springfield, Ill.: Charles C Thomas. 1969.
280. Zeligman, I., Hubener, L. F.: Experimental production of acne by progesterone. A.M.A. Arch. Derm. 76, 652—658 (1957).
281. Zielske, F., Dreykluft, R., Magnus, U., Hammerstein, J.: Reversed sequential therapy of hirsutism using cyproterone acetate. Acta endocr. Suppl. *152*, 15 (1971).
283. Zöllner, N., Kirsch, K.: Über die quantitative Bestimmung von Lipoiden. Z. ges. exp. Med. *135*, 545—557 (1962).